Borderline Personality Disorder

Tailoring the Psychotherapy to the Patient

Borderline Personality Disorder

Tailoring the Psychotherapy to the Patient

Leonard Horwitz, Ph.D.
Glen O. Gabbard, M.D.
Jon G. Allen, Ph.D.
Siebolt H. Frieswyk, Ph.D.
Donald B. Colson, Ph.D.
Gavin E. Newsom, M.S.W.
Lolafaye Coyne, Ph.D.

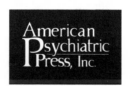

Washington, DC
London, England

Note: The authors have worked to ensure that all information in this book concerning drug dosages, schedules, and routes of administration is accurate as of the time of publication and consistent with standards set by the U.S. Food and Drug Administration and the general medical community. As medical research and practice advance, however, therapeutic standards may change. For this reason and because human and mechanical errors sometimes occur, we recommend that readers follow the advice of a physician who is directly involved in their care or the care of a member of their family.

Books published by the American Psychiatric Press, Inc., represent the views and opinions of the individual authors and do not necessarily represent the policies and opinions of the Press or the American Psychiatric Association.

Copyright © 1996 American Psychiatric Press, Inc.
ALL RIGHTS RESERVED
Manufactured in the United States of America on acid-free paper
99 98 97 96   4 3 2 1
First Edition

American Psychiatric Press, Inc.
1400 K Street, N.W., Washington, DC   20005

Library of Congress Cataloging-in-Publication Data
Borderline personality disorder : tailoring the psychotherapy to the
   patient / by Leonard Horwitz ... [et al.]. — 1st ed.
      p.   cm.
   Includes bibliographical references and index.
   ISBN 0-88048-689-9 (alk. paper)
   1. Borderline personality disorder—Treatment.   2. Psychiatry—
Differential therapeutics.   I. Horwitz, Leonard, 1922–   .
   [DNLM: 1. Borderline Personality Disorder—therapy.
2. Psychotherapy—methods.   WM 190B728935 1996]
RC569.5.B67B6894—1996
616.85'8520651—dc20
DNLM/DLC
for Library of Congress   95-36000
                                                                        CIP

British Library Cataloguing in Publication Data
A CIP record is available from the British Library.

Contents

Contributors

Jon G. Allen, Ph.D.
Senior Staff Psychologist, Trauma Recovery Program,
C. F. Menninger Memorial Hospital; and Editor, *Bulletin of the
Menninger Clinic,* Topeka, Kansas

Donald B. Colson, Ph.D.
Chief Psychologist, The Menninger Clinic; and Graduate, Topeka
Institute for Psychoanalysis, Topeka, Kansas

Lolafaye Coyne, Ph.D.
Director, Statistical Laboratory; and Acting Director, Research
Department, The Menninger Clinic, Topeka, Kansas

Siebolt H. Frieswyk, Ph.D.
Coordinator, Psychotherapy Training, Karl Menninger School of
Psychiatry and Mental Health Sciences; and Faculty Member,
Topeka Institute for Psychoanalysis, Topeka, Kansas

Glen O. Gabbard, M.D.
Bessie Walker Callaway Distinguished Professor of Psychoanalysis
and Education, Karl Menninger School of Psychiatry and Mental
Health Sciences; Training and Supervising Analyst, Topeka
Institute for Psychoanalysis, Topeka, Kansas; and Clinical
Professor of Psychiatry, University of Kansas School of
Medicine—Wichita, Wichita, Kansas

Leonard Horwitz, Ph.D.
Training and Supervising Analyst, Topeka Institute for
Psychoanalysis; Director, Treatment Interventions Project, The
Menninger Clinic, Topeka, Kansas; and Clinical Professor of
Psychiatry, University of Kansas School of Medicine—Wichita,
Wichita, Kansas

Gavin E. Newsom, M.S.W.
Chief Social Worker, The Menninger Clinic, Topeka, Kansas

Preface

Patients with borderline personality disorder comprise a large segment of the difficult-to-treat population. The instability of their relationships, the intensity of their affective responses, and their proneness to paranoid reactions all contribute to their difficulty in working consistently and constructively in the psychotherapeutic situation. When one adds to these difficult patient problems the therapist's quandary about how expressive or supportive to be, therapists are indeed often confronted with a challenging therapeutic task.

About a decade ago, a small group of senior clinicians at the Menninger Clinic decided to embark on a study of the psychotherapy of borderline patients. This population of personality disorders constituted a large segment of our patient group, both inpatient and outpatient. Our objective was not only to learn more about the issue of when to use supportive versus expressive methods, but to help improve moment-to-moment treatment interventions.

Early on we made certain strategic decisions. We made the assumption that borderline personality represents a broad spectrum of conditions and that the optimal intervention for one patient may be inappropriate for another. In addition to the different responses needed by different types of patients, we wished to understand how varying moods and anxieties influence the tactical decisions of the therapist.

We also decided early on that a desirable method of assessing the patient's reactions to therapeutic interventions, particularly the determination of the effectiveness of the therapist's responses, was to attempt to measure the shifts in the therapeutic alliance between patient and therapist. Our assumption was that the alliance would be a good barometer of how well the therapist was facilitating or hindering the ongoing work of the therapy.

To accomplish a microscopic, fine-grained study of the therapy process in which we learn more about how the therapist contributes to or hinders the therapeutic work, we deemed it necessary to record every psychotherapy session and to study a randomly selected group of sessions. Our hope was to provide the clinician with increased insight into what is most effective with what kind of patient at a given point in the therapy process.

The present work continues a long tradition of clinical research at the Menninger Clinic. Starting with the ground-breaking work on projective testing done by David Rapaport and his colleagues in the 1940s, and followed by one of the most ambitious studies of long-term psychotherapy ever executed—the Menninger Psychotherapy Research Project—Menninger has continuously supported studies designed to better understand our patients and the clinical work we do with them.

The study we are presenting is a spin-off of the earlier Psychotherapy Research Project. The senior author was involved in that work almost from its inception and had responsibility for the prediction study. His analysis of the data, as well as Wallerstein's comprehensive study, differed in some important respects from the study of the quantitative data done by Kernberg. The disagreement revolved around the effectiveness of supportive psychotherapy, particularly with patients with weak egos.

The above disagreement has been partially resolved by recent advances in understanding the nature of borderline pathology. In particular, Meissner has attempted to relate his concept of the continuum or spectrum of borderline illness to indications for varying degrees of supportiveness and expressiveness in treatment. A significant clinical question is no longer which form of treatment is better, but rather which modality or combination of modalities is most suitable for which type of borderline patients.

The rapid changes over the past few years in mental health care, particularly as it pertains to hospitalization, may lead to some questions about the treatment approach used with these patients. Two of our three patients were hospitalized for longer than a year—one because of the danger of suicide, and the other because of poorly controlled drug use and other self-damaging behaviors. The reader needs to take into account that these psychotherapy processes were recorded in an era in which extended hospital treatment was commonplace for borderline patients. Current health care policies regarding length of hospitalization would, for better or worse, oppose these lengthy hospitalizations for patients with severe character problems. We are also aware that other treatment modalities, such as pharmacotherapy, group therapy, family therapy, and dialectical behavior therapy, are all useful and effective with certain patients. Our focus only on individual psychodynamic psychotherapy represents our special interest and expertise.

It has been our good fortune to have had a research team of seven members who have worked productively together over the past decade on this study. Six of us are experienced psychoanalytic clinicians, and the seventh is a statistical and design consultant. Our sustained enthusiasm for this collaborative work was enhanced by the opportunity to share and exchange clinical insights derived from the study of recorded psychotherapy sessions. It was a rare and valuable professional experience to be able to have detailed discussions of "live" clinical material with a group of colleagues.

In Chapter 1, we present both the clinical and research literature pertaining to the treatment of borderline patients, particularly from the point of view of the controversy surrounding the use of expressive and supportive interventions. In Chapter 2, we deal with the concept of the therapeutic alliance and emphasize our rationale for the specific aspect of the alliance that we focused on (i.e., patient collaboration). We include an overview of the research method used in this study, the details of which can be found in the Appendixes for those readers who are research oriented. Chapters 3, 4, and 5 are primarily clinically oriented descriptions of the three patients in our study, their psychotherapy process, and outcome. In the interest of confidentiality, the write-ups were sufficiently disguised to prevent identification of the patient. Our final chapter is devoted to a summary of the overall results and major conclusions of the study.

Acknowledgments

In addition to the seven-member research team who executed this study, we enlisted the help of four senior clinicians who made certain additional ratings of the data. They were Drs. Patrick Dattore and Joel Nance, who worked on the prediction study, and Drs. Melvin Berg and Lisa Lewis, who assessed outcomes.

We owe a large debt of gratitude to The Menninger Clinic for its support of this project, and in particular to Dr. Cotter Hirschberg, Duane Swanson, and later Dr. W. Walter Menninger for their encouragement and willingness to subsidize our efforts. Dr. Herbert Spohn, Director of Research, was an important consultant and supporter of this project. The Fund for Psychoanalytic Research of the American Psychoanalytic Association also contributed to our financial support. The project's secretary, Jill Loomans, was invaluable in keeping our files in order and doing the tedious job of typing transcripts. Faye Schoenfeld assisted us in putting our manuscript into readable form.

The Expressive Versus
Supportive Controversy

S cores of books and hundreds of articles on the diagnosis and treatment of patients with borderline personality disorder have
flooded the literature over the past 10–15 years. These writings speak
both to the theoretical advances that have been achieved in understanding these patients as well as to the great difficulty and challenge
that they pose for the psychotherapist. Thanks largely to the contributions of numerous clinicians and theorists who have focused their
studies on the conflicts, defenses, and deficits of the first 2–3 years of
life, we have achieved a far better understanding of borderline psychopathology than was formerly available. These insights have made
it possible to undertake more definitive treatment than was done previously, because the challenges presented, although formidable, were
at least understandable.

Everyone agrees that borderline patients constitute a most challenging population to the psychotherapist. Many do not allow themselves to be treated, as indicated by several studies of dropout rates.
In the first study (Skodol et al. 1983), 67% dropped out in the first
3 months, and, in the second (Gunderson et al. 1989), 40%–50% within
the first 6 months. Skodol et al. found that the rate of early discontinuance was nearly twice the rate seen in a neurotic or other personality disorder group and more than four times the rate observed in a
schizophrenic group.

1

More recently, Stevenson and Meares (1992) reported a dropout rate of 16% in a study of 48 borderline patients, although they did not include in that figure the 11 patients who completed the evaluation and later dropped out or the 3 patients who were dismissed from the study for failure to keep three consecutive evaluation appointments. Yeomans et al. (1994) studied 36 female borderline patients and noted a 36% dropout rate by the end of 6 months.

Even when they remain in therapy, borderline patients may fare poorly. Low success rates are suggested in the report by Waldinger and Gunderson (1987), who initially approached approximately 25 staff members known to be interested in the practice of intensive psychotherapy with patients suffering from severe personality disorders, with the intention of obtaining and studying patients who had been successfully treated with intensive psychodynamic therapy. Although the majority of this group had treated several borderline patients, none of them deemed any of their treatment cases to be successful, and hence the investigators needed to cast a wider net in the community to find five subjects.

Borderline patients tax the skill and patience of the most experienced psychotherapist because their behavior, both within and outside the treatment situation, is often destructive and self-destructive as well as unreasonably demanding and exasperating. Their moods are quixotic and unpredictable, often making the treatment emotionally stormy, and they show an intense craving for closeness that is countered by basic mistrust. They present a challenge to the therapist in maintaining a stable working relationship.

One of the major difficulties presented by borderline patients is their tendency to oscillate between positive and negative ego states. Kernberg (1975) elucidated this characteristic as one of the manifestations of the basic splitting defense used by these patients. Fluctuating between idealization and devaluation, they frequently leave the therapist puzzled, if not bewildered, by the jolting shifts in mood and attitude. One borderline patient, for example, was unusually positive and receptive for most of a session, and the therapist felt both gratified and free in communicating his understandings of the issues she was presenting. He was able to explain why she characteristically experienced herself as exploited by her friends and colleagues and how her reluctance to depend on others made it difficult for her to permit herself to enjoy a mutually reciprocal relationship. Toward the end of the session, her expression darkened, and in a dramatic about-face, she informed the therapist that none of his observations were particularly helpful, she had no idea how she could put them to use, and most of what the therapist said was unclear in any case! In retrospect, the patient was reenacting with the therapist the very problem she had been presenting, but the sudden and dramatic shift in attitude illustrates a primary difficulty in dealing with borderline patients.

A related problem is the effect on the therapist of the patient's demeaning devaluations. This behavior is not only associated with defensive splitting, which leaves the patient's aggression relatively unmodulated, but it also may be understood in terms of excessive aggression that characterizes these patients. Furthermore, the mechanism of projective identification, in which the patient both projects a mental content on the therapist and attempts to elicit a response consistent with that content, contributes to the struggle the therapist experiences. One therapist, for example, received repeated barrages from his patient of how ineffective, unhelpful, and upsetting her sessions were with him. Despite his extensive clinical experience and his excellent clinical skills, the repeated attacks on his professional competence produced in him a genuine crisis of confidence that he was able to overcome only after a number of consultations with a colleague.

Plainly, borderline patients evoke intense countertransference, and the therapists' management of countertransference may make or break the treatment (Gabbard and Wilkinson 1994). Once again, the concept of projective identification has contributed to a better understanding of the patient-therapist interaction and how the affective intensity of a patient's behavior may lead to difficult countertransference responses. Without minimizing the therapist's own neurotic propensities, the raw, primitive, unmodulated projections of the patient may lead to intensely distressing reactions in therapists and to a decrease in their effectiveness.

Another facet of the difficulty with these patients is the problem of underdiagnosis. A long-standing observation concerns their relatively smooth functioning in structured situations as opposed to their regressive reactions in unstructured situations (such as projective tests, the psychoanalytic situation, and certain social interactions). It is not uncommon for clinicians to overestimate the ego strength of a patient on the basis of the patient's intellectual or occupational accomplishments. Many therapists have had to learn through sad experience the fallacy of confusing an advanced degree with mental health. The Menninger Psychotherapy Research Project (Horwitz 1974) provided numerous examples of patients who were underdiagnosed on that basis and whose treatment was incorrectly prescribed, usually in the direction of being more unstructured and expressive than the patient was able to tolerate. In fact, a special study of 16 borderline patients in the Menninger project revealed that half of them had been incorrectly diagnosed in the direction of overestimating their ego strength at the outset of treatment (L. Horwitz, D. B. Colson, and S. F. Frieswyk: "Issues in the Diagnosis and Treatment of Borderline Patients," unpublished manuscript, 1986).

The Expressive Versus Supportive Controversy

A plethora of theories and technical approaches to the treatment of *the* borderline patient contributes to the quandary of the clinical practitioner. The surveys of various approaches reveal a range from the most expressive (including psychoanalysis) to the most supportive (Horwitz 1985; Waldinger 1987). Embattled therapists not only have to contend with patients who present taxing behaviors, elicit intense countertransference reactions, and often are assessed healthier and stronger than they actually are, but in addition they must confront these clinical issues without the support of a clear, unambiguous set of theoretical views and technical recommendations.

The clinical literature is rife with disagreement about how to treat borderline patients. Recommendations range from classical psychoanalysis to modified psychoanalytic psychotherapy to a low-frequency, low-intensity supportive treatment (Horwitz 1985; Waldinger 1987). Although some writers (Kernberg 1984; Masterson 1976) acknowledge there may be exceptional cases who do not qualify for their recommended treatment, others (Abend et al. 1983; Adler 1985; Volkan 1987) tend to present their views as though the borderline condition is relatively homogeneous and their approach is applicable across the board. Historically, the field began with a cautious, low-key, supportive approach in view of the predisposition to chaotic transferences and difficulties in forming a stable working alliance such patients demonstrate. As the pioneering work of theorists like Kernberg began to elucidate the underlying etiologies and defensive configurations of these patients, clinicians became emboldened to work more actively and intensively. The supportive versus expressive controversy, however, still persists.

Expressive treatment is defined as a therapy that attempts to explore and uncover the patient's unconscious wishes, fears, conflicts, and defenses. The most potent means of achieving the goal of making the unconscious conscious is to explore the underlying difficulties in relationships, particularly the patient's relationship to the therapist.

Supportive treatment is defined as a therapy in which the activities of the therapist-analyst promote the patient's adaptive functioning both within and outside of the therapeutic interaction. The therapist's actions that facilitate the patient's functioning include the use of the person of the therapist as a source of emotional support, affirming adaptive behavior. Equally important, the therapist functions as a model for identification in which the therapist's reality testing, judgment, anticipation of consequences, emotional constraint, and appropriateness, as well as other ego functions, guide and structure the patient.

Early Views

The concept of borderline personality began gaining attention in the early 1950s, and a fairly uniform viewpoint prevailed for the next two decades. Knight (1954) was typical of most dynamic theorists of that era who believed that the ego weakness of these patients was relatively irreversible. These patients were seen as prone to ego regressions under stress, often of psychotic proportions, and in need of a supportive approach that emphasized a strengthening of defenses. Uncovering unconscious transference reactions was to be avoided; rather, a reality-oriented approach was necessary to strengthen reality testing and enhance adaptive behavior.

Similarly, Zetzel (1971) was a strong proponent of this relatively conservative approach. Because she was impressed with the proneness of borderline patients to exhibit impulsive and regressive behavior and transferences that tended to be chaotic and primitive, Zetzel rec-

ommended that the therapist attempt to avoid any approach that could
intensify the transference. She called for infrequent therapy sessions,
not to exceed once a week, and she suggested a high degree of activity
and structured sessions to discourage the development of strong transference wishes or fears.

Use of Psychoanalysis

If Knight's conservative early approach represents one extreme, unmodified psychoanalysis is the other. A prominent departure from
the early views of Knight (1954) and Zetzel (1971), and to some extent from the prevailing current views, is the use of a more-or-less
classical psychoanalytic technique with borderline patients. Some
writers (Abend et al. 1983; Meissner 1984) think in terms of applying
psychoanalysis to a limited group of high-level borderline patients,
whereas others (Volkan 1987) recommend analysis (with the introduction of some parameters) even with psychosis-prone patients. Although relatively little has been written explicitly about standard
psychoanalysis with borderline individuals except by a small minority of writers, Waldinger and Gunderson (1984) polled a group of clinicians who had extensive experience in the long-term treatment of
these patients and who themselves had made significant contributions to the literature regarding their experiences with such cases.
The 11 therapists who participated, of 30 who were invited, reported
the surprising result that in the sample of 78 patients whose treatments were described, more than half (59%) were treated in psychoanalysis, and the rest were treated in intensive psychotherapy. Of
course, these were not run-of-the-mill therapists, and most pertinent
was that 10 of the 11 had had psychoanalytic training.

Abend et al. (1983) studied four patients who underwent psychoanalysis with psychoanalytic candidates. Two of them fit the criteria
of borderline personality organization as described by Kernberg
(1975); the other two were viewed as within the neurotic range according to the Kernberg criteria. The feasibility of an intensive psychoanalytic procedure with these patients, with a minimum of
parameters, fits with Meissner's (1984, 1988) view that the borderline
spectrum from high-level to low-level functioning patients includes
a group at the high end who may be amenable to psychoanalysis. In

his preanalytic assessment, Meissner attempts to discern reasonable levels of ego functioning—the ability to withstand frequent and intensive pulls, consistent and realistic levels of motivation, and most important, a capacity for forming and maintaining a reasonably stable therapeutic alliance.

The experience of the Menninger Psychotherapy Research Project in using psychoanalysis to treat borderline patients was almost uniformly negative (Horwitz 1974). Retrospective judgments at the end of treatment about the suitability of each case for analysis revealed that 10 patients (about 50%) were seen as unsuitable for an analytic procedure. Six of those patients manifested borderline personality organizations with a potential for psychotic reactions and reacted with delusional thinking, either within the transference or in their life situations. One patient who showed borderline features was successfully treated. In evaluating this finding, the context of these treatments must be considered. They mainly occurred in the latter part of the 1950s when the strong prevailing view in psychoanalysis was against the use of a regression-inducing treatment for patients with ego weaknesses. In addition, many of these patients had been underdiagnosed initially, and therefore the regressive potential and the ego disorganization that they evidenced during the analytic process was unexpected and viewed as an unwelcome development. Finally, the understanding of borderline pathology that has developed since that time, particularly in the area of advances in object relations theory and in developmental theory, was not available to the analysts of that period.

A small band of devoted workers, often imbued with a sense of mission and with intense conviction, have been striving without great success to convince their psychoanalytic colleagues that even the quite regressed borderline patients, those who are psychosis-prone, are able to benefit from a standard psychoanalytic procedure (Boyer 1977; Giovacchini 1979; Volkan 1987). They believe that the sine qua non of treating borderline disorders is a therapeutic regression to the level of the patient's conflict-based fixations to permit the dissolution of archaic, maladaptive introjects and the beginning growth and acquisition of new ones. Volkan reported on his work with nine psychosis-prone patients who were seen in psychoanalysis four to five times per week with an average length of treatment of 6 years. He used the couch after the first phase of treatment, which has the aim of establishing a reality base and a core therapeutic alliance. All his patients showed "drastic improvement," although two were somewhat less successful than the others in that they did not resolve their primitive unconscious conflicts, nor did they move up to an oedipal level.

Volkan (1987) contrasted his approach with those who attempted to support patients at a level where they can function without further regression, a basically supportive approach; surprisingly, he suggested that Kernberg (1975) falls into this category. He believed that Kernberg tried to effect a fusion of split self- and object-representations without the benefit of a transference psychosis. These splits are integrated by Kernberg's use of clarification, interpretation, and confrontation (in particular, his confrontations with contradictory ego attitudes), but the loop consisting of therapeutic regression is bypassed. Unquestionably, Volkan's approach is more intensive and regression inducing than the leading methods to be reported here. We concur with the majority opinion that unmodified psychoanalysis is indicated for only a very limited group of high-level borderline patients.

Expressive-Interpretive Approaches

Kernberg's (1975, 1976) important contributions to our understanding of the early developmental conflicts that lead to borderline psychopathology have made it more feasible than before to consider using an intensive and interpretive approach. He elucidated borderline patients' difficulty in accomplishing the developmental task of dealing with Mahler et al.'s (1975) rapprochement stage and hence has been unable to move beyond the use of primitive splitting as described by Melanie Klein (1946/1975). Like Klein, Kernberg subscribed to the view that the major psychological conflict for borderline patients is the management of intense aggression, based partly on constitutional factors and partly on the predominance of aggression over libido in the child's early experiences.

Thus, in Kernberg's (1976) view, the therapist must be alert for evidence of negative transference early on and interpret it actively whenever it appears. Failure to do so will lead to the negative transference going underground, resulting in a buildup of aggression that could either cause a rupture of the alliance or eventuate in a distant, stalemated relationship.

Kernberg (1984) recognized that his expressive-interpretive approach requires modification because borderline patients behave impulsively in destructive and self-destructive ways and are capable of threatening the treatment or their life situation when sufficient treatment parameters are not introduced. For example, the initial contract with the patient should include provisions for what limits the therapist will impose if the patient behaves destructively (Kernberg et al. 1989). Also, Kernberg favored using external supports (ranging from counselors to hospitalization) for those patients who are unable to structure their lives by themselves. He suggested that deviations from the stance of technical neutrality be used, however sparingly, to control acting out.

Initially, Kernberg (1976) emphasized one major contraindication to expressive psychotherapy with borderline patients—those patients with prominent narcissistic character pathology who would be given to attacks of narcissistic rage when experiencing frustration or criticism from the therapist. Later, Kernberg (1984) expanded his list of contraindications to include the following: 1) hypomanic personalities and as-if personalities with "pseudologia fantastica," the latter because of the tendency toward lying; 2) severe forms of negative therapeutic reactions in which the patient identifies with an extremely sadistic, primitive object; 3) patients who are alcoholic, drug addicted, or chronically suicidal; 4) chaotic life circumstances; 5) a chronic absence of actual object relations or marked social isolation; and 6) the presence of severe nonspecific manifestations of ego weakness. If the patient's illness is providing a substantial degree of secondary gain, the prognosis for expressive psychotherapy is not good.

Although other writers (Abend et al. 1983; Chessick 1982; Gunderson 1984; Masterson 1976; Meissner 1988) have subscribed to the idea of intensive work with borderline individuals, none is as ready to begin this work as early nor with as much vigor as Kernberg. The exceptions may be Boyer (1977), Giovacchini (1979), and Volkan (1987), as previously described, but even they believed in a slow-paced approach at the beginning. Masterson (1976) recommended an active reconstructive method for those borderline patients who can tolerate such work, but his approach differed from Kernberg's in some important respects. Masterson believed that treatment must start with a relatively slow-paced "testing" phase, lasting for months or even years, in which the therapist works with the patient's initial resistances and focuses on establishing a therapeutic alliance by primarily supportive methods (i.e., the therapist's consistency, commitment, and trustworthiness).

Some patients, however, may not have the capacity to move beyond this initial stage, and Masterson (1976) noted the following contraindications to intensive treatment: 1) patients who have experienced repetitive and massive trauma in the crucial separation-individuation phase; 2) patients who show distancing rather than clinging as a predominant relationship mode; and 3) those who are closer to the psychotic level, who show strong paranoid features or intermittent psychotic episodes. Another major difference is that even in the interpretive stage of treatment, therapeutic neutrality is not consistently maintained and is not regarded as an important therapeutic position. Masterson focused on the split between being rewarded by an internal mother figure for remaining symbiotically attached to her, as opposed to the expectation of mother's withdrawal when the patient attempts to separate, with an ensuing abandonment depression. This conflict must be consistently interpreted and worked through, but in doing so, the therapist should actively take the role of the parent who encourages separation and achievement. Praise is freely given, congratulating the patient for progress made and, through "communicative matching" in which the therapist inquires into the details of the patient's work and interests, he or she reinforces the patient's growth. Thus, Kernberg's (1975) approach of expressive psychotherapy stands in contrast to Masterson's more mixed supportive-expressive treatment.

Gunderson (1984) also espoused an intensive approach but with the important caveat that this method should be attempted only by well-trained therapists working in an environment where hospitalization is available. He has taken a middle position between Kernberg and Masterson with regard to the technical aspects of interpretive treatment. On the issue of early interpretation of the negative transference, he believed that such behavior should be addressed and explored when overt and manifest, without necessarily being uncovered and interpreted. Interpretation, in Gunderson's view, should be used only when the patient's level of anxiety and sense of relatedness to the therapist permit the patient to understand and use the therapist's interpretation. The therapist must assess whether the patient feels sufficiently supported by and involved in the therapy, a precondition for offering interpretations. Finally, he believed, like Masterson (1976), that the therapist should provide the patient with a corrective emotional experience by trying to encourage and reinforce the patient's movement toward more adaptive and more mature behavior.

Kolb and Gunderson (1990) challenged Kernberg's (1975) designation of his psychotherapeutic approach as "expressive." They pointed out that a therapy that relies so heavily on limit setting and confrontation and places free association in such a subordinate role is far from expressive. In critiquing Kernberg et al.'s (1989) book, Kolb and Gunderson also questioned Kernberg's conceptualization that the patient's pathology is projected onto a "blank-screen" therapist. They noted the extensive correcting, explaining, warning, limit setting, problem solving, and educating that is characteristic of Kernberg's style of psychotherapy and suggested that these provocative departures from neutrality should be considered as powerful stimulants for patients' reactions. Gunderson and Kolb also suggested that Kernberg and his collaborators were biased against the notion of supportive therapy even though there were clearly supportive elements in their approach. Gunderson's (1984) view of borderline psychopathology revolved around the patient's anxiety concerning separation from the "primary object" (parents, spouse, therapist) and how the patient's symptoms and pathological behavior get mobilized by the loss, or threat of loss, of these objects.

In summary, Kernberg (1975) emphasized adherence as much as possible to an interpretive approach from the position of neutrality, eschewing supportive measures wherever possible. Masterson (1976) recommended a slower approach to interpretive techniques and endorsed the idea of support for adaptive change. Gunderson (1984) took something of a middle course between these two, arguing for a careful assessment of the patient's readiness to deal with interpretive uncovering work, but at the same time joined Masterson in emphasizing the importance of supporting the patient's movement and growth. Those who advocate an expressive approach do not do so without reservation. The views about contraindications for uncovering interpretive work were varied, but may be summarized as follows.

1. Patients who had undergone traumatic experiences of loss and separation could not tolerate exploratory work, presumably because it threatened the loss of an idealized therapeutic relationship.
2. Patients who were distant and paranoid, as opposed to dependent and clinging, would tend to hear interpretive comments as critical and accusatory.
3. Patients who had poor impulse control were prone to engage in destructive and self-destructive acting out in reaction to the increased anxiety associated with interpretive work.
4. Narcissistic patients who experienced any nonaffirming intervention as a threat to their tenuous sense of self-esteem would become distant or enraged.

Supportive Approaches

The major writers who have formulated borderline pathology as based on a developmental defect associated with inadequate parenting are Adler (1985), Buie and Adler (1982/1983), and Chessick (1977). Adler's ideas closely follow the writings of Kohut (1977) in viewing borderline patients as suffering from a failure to develop soothing-holding introjects; hence, they are hypersensitive to frustration, loss, and a sense of aloneness, which in turn lead to regressed chaotic behavior and acting out. In contrast to conflict theorists, these clinicians believed that the primary curative factor is the patient's experience of being symbolically held and soothed by the therapist, compensating for the deficient parenting experiences of early development. This view of borderline pathology leads to important technical differences with a conflict theorist like Kernberg.

To the extent that interpretations are used early in treatment, the emphasis is on uncovering the idealization of the therapist, which often tends to be defended against by aloofness and devaluation. In contrast, Adler (1985) emphasized the importance of confronting the patient with various aspects of reality (i.e., continued existence of the therapist as a caring object who does not resemble the hostile introjects that the patient projects and dangerous situations that the patient minimizes or denies). Although accepting Kernberg's (1975) view of the need to heal the long-standing split between the good and bad self and object representations, Adler believed that such efforts must be postponed until a stable holding introject has been established. Like Kohut (1977), he theorized that rage reactions are the product of empathic failure and that interpretive activity largely deals with transference frustrations and parental failures.

Supportive measures include limit setting on the behavior within the session and structuring the interview, as well as showing overt gestures of care and concern. Adler (1985) stated that "transitional objects (for example, vacation addresses and postcards), extra appointments, and telephone calls reaffirming that the therapist exists are required at various times, and, for the more severely borderline personalities, one or two brief hospitalizations may be expected" (p. 52). The major emphasis is on the patient's experience rather than the content, on providing soothing-holding figures to internalize, rather than insight into conflicts. Because the treatment approach emphasizes support, the method seems to be applicable to a wide range of borderline subtypes and levels of ego functioning, in contrast to a more strictly interpretive approach that may be used only with those patients who have the ego resources to tolerate an uncovering process. Adler did, however, emphasize that borderline patients with strong narcissistic vulnerabilities need to have "definitive treatment" delayed until the latter phases of treatment when a firm holding figure has been internalized.

Chessick (1979) advocated a slow, gradual approach in dealing with the patient's transferences. In his view, those patients who show Kohut's mirroring or idealizing transference, whereby the therapist is seen as an extension of the self, should ideally be permitted to hold on to these transferences until they are ready to drop away spontaneously. These patients require a symbiotic, fused relationship with the therapist, at least in the early stages, and should not be pressured to alter the relationship until they show signs of being ready to do so on their own. On the other hand, Chessick believed that an intense negative or erotized transference needs to be addressed early by interpretation or confrontation in which the discrepancy between what the patient is experiencing and the reality of the treatment situation is pointed out and explored. Chessick recognized that doing this early in the therapy relationship, when a therapeutic alliance has still not been formed, presents a difficult and potentially disruptive problem.

He distinguished between the narcissistic and transitional object transferences as opposed to disruptive transferences and felt that the former need to be left alone and permitted to "drop away by themselves" whereas the latter need confrontation.

One extension of the self psychological viewpoint is the intersubjective perspective. Brandchaft and Stolorow (1987) claimed that Kernberg's (1975) concept of borderline personality organization is "largely, if not entirely, an iatrogenic myth" (p. 124). In their view, defining the borderline phenomenon as residing solely in the patient is inaccurate. Rather, such phenomena occur in an intersubjective field consisting of a patient with a vulnerable and precarious self combined with a failing, archaic selfobject that may be a therapist or other person in the environment. Operating from this assumption, Brandchaft and Stolorow suggested that borderline symptoms appear when the therapist fails to appreciate the patient's selfobject needs. They argued that to divorce the clinical phenomena of borderline personality disorder from the intersubjective context in which they arise is artificial and invalid. Although making a valid point regarding the importance of the therapist's input, their view appears to de-emphasize the ego weaknesses that exist in people independent of their surround.

Specific Technical Considerations

There are a group of writers who are not easily categorized into the supportive or expressive camp but who, nevertheless, have proposed specific treatment ideas that deserve careful consideration. Some point to common pitfalls in analytic therapy; others offer special techniques in dealing with this population of borderline patients.

Epstein (1979), for example, emphasized the noxious effects of an active interpretive approach and instead recommended a slower-paced method of "containing, reflecting, and investigating." His thesis was that the typical defense of borderline patients is projecting or externalizing unacceptable aspects of the self and that this defense needs to be relinquished gradually as the patient experiences a decreasing need for it. Epstein contended that the most serious mistake a therapist can make with the patient who is projecting negative aspects of the self (e.g., stupidity, badness, unattractiveness) onto the therapist is to interpret the patient's defensive projection. Rather, patients must become aware only gradually that such feelings are a part of their own self-image, and this awareness will occur in the context of the growing safety of the therapeutic relationship and the increasing ability to face their less acceptable parts.

Meissner (1982) held a similar point of view and provided a careful rationale for working slowly and systematically, rather than interpretively, with paranoid patients. The patients' projections are rooted in their system of introjects, and those introjects can be examined only after a gradual and painstaking examination of the reality of the projections. Meissner described the technique of "tagging," in which the therapist emphasizes the difference between the patient's feelings or inferences and the actual events. He also recommended the need to clarify those situations in which gaps in knowledge weaken the patient's conclusions. As the conviction about the validity of the projections begins to weaken, the patient's introjective system can be examined.

Pine (1984) offered the unique perspective that the special ego defects of the "seriously disturbed" patient need to be recognized, and interpretations should be timed and modified so that the vulnerable ego of the patient can be supported as much as possible. He made a series of recommendations regarding how and when interpretations should be offered in such a way as to minimize the patient's discomfort (e.g., "strike when the iron is cold"). Thus, in addition to the interpretive content, therapists ought to convey explicitly that they are not about to abandon their patients and that they will persevere with them no matter how often the maladaptive behavior is repeated. Pine also recommended taking steps to counteract the patient's usual inclination to lapse into passivity in the process of listening and reacting to an interpretation as a result of dependency and idealizing tendencies. He further advised that the therapist provide a holding environment while offering an interpretation. Rather than polarize interpretive therapy and supportive therapy, one should distinguish between "interpretation given within the context of abstinence," which characterizes classical analysis, and "interpretation given within the context of support," which characterizes Pine's recommendations for working with disturbed patients. This new conceptualization tends to shift the supportive-expressive issue from an either/or problem into a more inclusive both/and mode of thinking and holds promise for expanding the indications for interpretive work.

Schaffer (1986) took a similar approach to that of Pine (1984) in that he recommended the so-called affirmative interpretation. Schaffer believed that the mode of interpreting, not interpreting per se, is the critical feature of expressive work. The ideal approach would be to offer interpretations and confrontations within the context of emphasizing the adaptive value of the patient's behavior, so that the confrontation of splitting, for example, would include observations regarding the patient's attempt to maintain a good relationship with someone. Also, Schaffer stressed the importance of including an empathic comment regarding the struggles and reasons for a particular kind of maladaptive behavior.

All these writers have addressed themselves to the proneness to narcissistic injury in the borderline patient population and their need to externalize and project. More recently, several other articles have appeared that focus on the danger of early confrontations. Gunderson et al. (1989) studied early dropouts and concluded that a major factor contributing to premature terminations was too much early confrontation. They found that more than half of the clinical dropouts left in anger after early confrontation with their problems, underscoring the brittle sensitivity and relative intolerance of many borderline patients for the usual demands and common frustrations of psychotherapy. The importance of supportive techniques early in the therapy process was emphasized.

Gabbard (1991) made a similar point with regard to the subgroup of borderline patients who use projective identification to disavow aspects of the hated internal world and project them into the analyst. The result is a relentless transference hatred that is unresponsive to interpretation. Treatment becomes threatened by the possible erosion of the analyst's ability to maintain a sound analytic stance. What is necessary in such circumstances is a suitably long period of containment, as opposed to active interpretation or confrontation, to permit both analyst and patient sufficient time to integrate the intensely negative feelings with more positive affects to regain the capacity to process analytic experiences in a reflective "analytic space."

The consensus in all these observations is that, in dealing with patients who "hate" (those who manifest a predominance of paranoid pathology), analytic therapists need to process their own counter-transference retaliatory hate. Ideally, one should be able to contain the patient's aggression without either masochistically submitting or sadistically attacking. Although Epstein (1979) generally adopted this stance, he believed that there is a special subcategory of such patients who need to have their negativity interrupted by the therapist. He distinguished between patients whose destructiveness is reactive rather than malevolent, that is, those who "enter treatment primed with a strong unconscious intention to destroy it" (p. 392). Epstein characterized these patients as exhibiting a malignant process in which they attempt an "insidious penetration of the analyst's boundaries with the aim of destroying, maiming, poisoning or otherwise damaging his insides" (p. 392). Such patients need an openly aggressive response from the analyst of sufficient intensity to reestablish the self-other boundaries and hopefully to reengage the patient's reasonable ego. The kind of diagnostic differentiation implied in this observation (reactive versus malevolent) is an important distinction requiring further work.

Research Perspectives on Intensive Psychotherapy

Several formal research studies have appeared in the recent past that throw light on supportive versus expressive treatment approaches with borderline patients. These projects vary from the intensive study of a few cases done by a number of outside judges who based their conclusions on consensus judgments, to a large-scale formal study in which a variety of objective instruments and rating scales were used to assess the patients and their therapy.

The earliest formal investigation on this subject was the quantitative study of the Menninger Psychotherapy Research Project. Kernberg et al. (1972) reported the finding that borderline patients receiving supportive treatment did not fare as well as those receiving a more expressively oriented therapy. Kernberg et al. based their report solely on the quantitative and statistical data of the project and were handicapped by not including the rich qualitative data describing the details of the patients and their treatment. Two other members of the project (Horwitz 1974; Wallerstein 1986) examined all the available research data, both qualitative and quantitative, and arrived at a conclusion that contradicted Kernberg et al.'s findings. They both observed that a predominantly supportive treatment was indeed effective with patients who showed weak egos and that these patients benefited from this approach to a much greater extent than expected. One should note, however, that the treatments in this project were administered mainly in the latter part of the 1950s, when the accepted modality for borderline patients was supportive therapy. Hence, there was no real opportunity to assess how these same patients might have fared with a more intensive approach.

Abend et al. (1983) reported on the study of four borderline patients who had been in psychoanalysis with psychoanalytic candidates for which detailed notes of the process were available. Clearly high-level borderline patients who could tolerate the analytic procedure, they did not require hospitalization at any time. When Kernberg studied these cases as part of his consultation with Abend's research group, he stated that two of the four patients met his criteria for borderline personality organization. The team's conclusion was that this particular group of patients was analyzable and could be treated by a relatively unmodified analytic method, although offering a special challenge to the analysts by virtue of their ego weakness characterized by projective thinking and impulsive behavior. Abend et al. contended that "no special techniques need be recommended for the analysis of borderline patients" (p. 200). Obviously, their conclusions apply to a narrow range of the borderline spectrum.

Waldinger and Gunderson (1987) intensively studied five borderline patients who were successfully treated by a group of experienced, analytically oriented therapists. Although the range of therapeutic techniques varied considerably within and among the five treatments, the general tendency was toward an initial period of acceptance and alliance building with a gradual movement toward increasing confrontation and limit setting. All the treatments were characterized by an unusually strong commitment by the therapists to persevere at the work until a satisfactory outcome was achieved, and this was an important factor contributing to the eventual development of strong alliances in each case. Whether the development of the alliance was due to interpretive efforts in the early stages of treatment was not clear, but confrontation and limit setting in the later stages of treatment were clearly helpful. Likewise, encouraging patients to express their anger toward the therapist and the therapist's nonretaliatory acceptance helped to strengthen the alliance. A major observation of the study was that none of the five patients was manifestly diagnosable as borderline after 4 years of treatment. Unfortunately, the study did not focus on the issue of what kind of borderline patients are more amenable or less amenable to interpretive techniques.

Stone's (1990) extensive follow-up study of more than 500 hospitalized patients, most of whom were borderline, examined the issue of the effectiveness of supportive and expressive techniques with this population. First, he attempted a controlled experiment with a small subsample of patients who initially seemed suitable for expressive psychotherapy and who were assigned to a particular ward where they were randomly given either supportive or expressive treatment. The same second-year residents did both treatments, and in comparing six patients in each category, no statistically significant differences in outcome were found. Stone acknowledged important flaws in this experiment, not the least of which was the relative inexperience of the therapists.

Stone (1990) also examined the treatments of 50 patients who fell into the category of successful outcomes, and at least 10 of these were highly insightful and motivated people who could work well with transference themes and dreams. He believed that the expressive psychotherapy these patients received not only facilitated their recovery, but enhanced their maturation and their eventual life adjustment. On the other hand, expressive psychotherapy proved too difficult for a number of borderline patients. In particular, Stone singled out those who tended to develop erotic transferences, were incest victims, had been repeatedly attacked by a parent, lost one or both parents through suicide, or were inordinately fragile or clinging.

Looking at his sample as a whole, Stone (1990) determined that between one-seventh and one-third of the sample benefited from expressive psychotherapy. Certain groups of patients were obviously excluded from treatment by an expressive modality: schizophrenic patients, seriously addicted patients, eating disorder patients, patients with affective comorbidity, unmotivated patients, as well as several other types. Many borderline patients did as well with some supportive forms of treatment, even a period of sanctuary in the hospital, as they did with expressive treatment. He recognized that because the therapists were in the early stages of training, many did not have the requisite skills to deal with this difficult population. Stone concluded that he was "prepared to believe that the dynamic/interpretive aspects of expressive therapy may have more specific value for a subgroup of ambulatory borderline patients, who eventually rise to adaptive heights they might not have reached with supportive psychotherapy" (p. 272).

Finally, a study by Piper et al. (1991) was not confined to borderline patients but included the related variable of high and low quality of object relations. The project involved 64 patients who had completed 20 once-a-week therapy sessions, the planned amount, with experienced psychodynamic therapists using a method of brief therapy modeled according to Malan (1976) as well as Strupp and Binder (1984). The variables of percentage of transference interpretation and quality of object relations were measured. Patients with a *high* quality of object relations responded poorly to a high frequency of transference interpretations (more than one-fifth). Piper's group explained that interpretive work tended to be overdone and that "there was too much of a good thing." No relationship between percentage of transference of interpretations and outcome for patients with a *low* quality of object relations was noted. The inconsistency within the group with low quality of object relations fits with the general observation that some borderline patients respond best to expressive methods whereas others respond best to supportive methods. An important omission in their study is the assessment of the adequacy (e.g., accuracy, timing, tact) of the transference interpretations.

Types of Borderline Patients

The wide divergence of viewpoints in treating borderline patients may be largely understood in terms of the broad spectrum encompassing this diagnostic category. Thus, in comparing the expressive-interpretive approach of Kernberg (1975) with the slower paced, more supportive recommendation of Adler (1979), Gunderson (1984) proposed the explanation that Kernberg's experience was based essentially on a setting where a hospital was readily available as opposed to Adler's work, which was based primarily on an outpatient setting. This difference in setting contributes to the differences between the two in the types of patients they treated. Whereas Kernberg's prototypical borderline patients were angry and impulsive, Adler's patients were more often described as depressed and withdrawn. Borderline personality disorder is obviously not a discrete, homogeneous entity and comprises a wide range of ego structures, pathological defenses, and character types. The thicket of proposed treatments may be disentangled and clarified by finding the correct therapeutic approach for the specific type of borderline patient.

All writers recognize that the category of borderline personality disorder embraces patients who range from functioning close to a neurotic level to those bordering on psychosis. The numerous books and articles on the treatment of borderline patients have often attempted to ignore these variations and have offered treatment prescriptions and manuals from the standpoint of the modal patient the authors have tended to select or work with. Nevertheless, a few writers have attempted to delineate specific borderline subtypes, with or without the intention of offering differential treatment strategies.

Grinker et al. (1968) were among the first workers to do an empirical study of the borderline syndrome. They found four types that they described as follows: Group 1, closest to the psychotic border, has given up attempts at developing relationships and overtly reacts negatively and angrily toward others. Group 2, representing the core process of the borderline group, was inconsistent in moving toward and away from others and characteristically made efforts to form relationships, but these were usually followed by withdrawal and isolation accompanied by feelings of loneliness and depression. Group 3, the as-if type, was mainly characterized by a marked weakness of identity and an effort to please and ingratiate as a defense against separation and abandonment. Finally, group 4, closest to the neurotic border, was characterized by a search for a lost symbiotic union with mother that constantly eludes them, resulting in an anaclitic depression.

More recently, Hurt and Clarkin (1990), members of the Kernberg research group, proposed a three-cluster model of borderline subtypes based on a study of 465 individuals, both inpatient and outpatient, who were assigned the DSM-III-R (American Psychiatric Association 1987) diagnosis of borderline personality disorder. The first was an *identity* cluster characterized by a chronic sense of emptiness, boredom, identity disturbance, and intolerance of being alone. These patients had an intense need for involvement with others and relied on external support for self-definition. Second was the *affective* cluster, who tended to show intense and inappropriate anger, instability of affect, and unstable relationships, mainly because of their propensity for stormy and intense affective reactions. Third was the *impulse* cluster, those who were prone to impulsive self-destructive behavior and who tended to show both life- and treatment-threatening behavior. Although these clusters showed some similarity to the Grinker et al. (1968) subtypes, no effort was made to include differentiations with regard to degree of pathology.

The most detailed and comprehensive effort to date to formulate borderline subtypes was done by Meissner (1984) in his excellent volume, *The Borderline Spectrum*. First, he introduced the notion that the divergent theoretical approaches to understanding borderline patients may, in fact, reflect the existence of "subvariants of pathological expression, which may be diagnostically differentiable" (p. 63). Taking this idea seriously, Meissner next proposed two broad continua, the hysterical and the schizoid, each having four subtypes along the borderline spectrum, ranging from most severe to least severe degrees of pathology, and he modestly proposed them as starting points for further investigation. The common factor among these subtypes is the underlying dilemma between a simultaneous need for and fear of involvement with objects.

The *hysterical* continuum consists of the following four subtypes: pseudoschizophrenia, psychotic character, dysphoric personality, and primitive hysteria. These are characterized by symbiotic needs and fantasies within an ego structure that varies from relatively undifferentiated (the pseudoschizophrenic and close to the psychotic border) to greater structuralization of introjects and stability of ego organization (the primitive hysteric, close to the neurotic border).

Meissner described the four points on the *schizoid* continuum as schizoid character, false-self organization, as-if personality, and identity stasis. The schizoid personality, close to the psychotic border, has a symbiotic wish for union with the object with the implication of symbiotic engulfment. The identity-stasis patients, with the highest level of organization, have major struggles in committing themselves to a decisive life course and embracing an authentic sense of identity.

In his subsequent volume, Meissner (1988) related each of his diagnostic subgroupings to particular therapeutic approaches. His line of thinking represents a significant departure from the "lumping" strategy proposed by many writers who basically adopt one therapeutic strategy for their modal type of borderline patients. His perspective is entirely consistent with the view of our research group that the choice of therapeutic modality, be it psychoanalysis or supportive psychotherapy, depends on an accurate assessment of the type of borderline patient being treated.

Summary of Indications and Contraindications for Expressive Work

Most writers, with the possible exception of Kernberg, recommend a slow-paced beginning in doing expressive psychotherapy with borderline patients. These patients need time to develop a sense of bonding and trust in the therapist's reliability and benevolence toward them before they are ready to engage in the process of uncovering aspects of their functioning that they have attempted to keep out of awareness. A new trend has developed over the years, however. Pine's (1984) "interpretation within the context of support" represents an effort to extend interpretive techniques as far as possible with borderline patients by recognizing their ego weaknesses and adjusting one's mix of interventions to accommodate the patient's special needs. Moreover, Gunderson (1984) emphasized the cogent point that expressive treatment with borderline patients ought to be attempted only by well-trained therapists (or at least well-supervised ones) who have an inpatient facility available as a backup resource.

The foregoing survey of the literature has yielded a rich harvest of variables that need to be considered before undertaking an expressive approach. They may be subsumed under three main rubrics: developmental factors, ego factors, and relationship factors. We now summarize the views that exist for each variable, and we use this conceptual framework based on the presented literature to examine the suitability of each of our three cases for expressive versus supportive interventions.

Developmental Factors

Early trauma.   Several writers have emphasized that repetitive and massive separation trauma during the separation-individuation phase tends to foreclose expressive work, presumably because the patient is usually oriented toward maintaining a close, symbiotic relationship with the therapist while interpretive work tends to emphasize their separateness.

Incest victims.   The trauma of betrayal, exploitation, and abuse often leaves incest victims unwilling to trust the therapist with intimate details of their lives. Hence, these patients need to maintain a psychological distance that is incompatible with expressive work.

Neurological dysfunction.   One study of borderline adolescents (Andrulonis et al. 1981) detected significant neurological dysfunctions, including episodic dyscontrol, seizure disorders, histories of head trauma, and minimal brain dysfunction. These investigators suggested that organic insults in childhood or genetic factors may play a key role in the etiology and pathogenesis of borderline personality disorder. More recently, four different studies of borderline patients have documented neuropsychological test abnormalities (Carpenter et al. 1993; Cornelius et al. 1989; Judd and Ruff 1993; O'Leary et al. 1991). Deficits were particularly noted in visuospatial skills and memory. There also appear to be specific problems in visual filtering and discrimination. The neuropsychological impairments are not obvious and may become apparent only when borderline patients are compared with a healthy control group (O'Leary and Cowdry 1994). Patients with these impairments lack the psychological-mindedness and capacity for abstraction and symbolic thinking necessary for expressive work.

Ego Factors

Unquestionably, the major consideration in deciding on the treatment of choice needs to be the diagnostic consideration of where the patient falls along the spectrum of borderline conditions going from high level (close to neurosis) versus low level (close to psychosis). The determination of where the patient lies along this continuum depends on the assessment of reality testing, impulse control, and degree of destructiveness and self-destructiveness, including suicidality. Although recognizing that severe deficiencies in ego capacities and controls may contraindicate expressive work, Kernberg (1976) relied heavily on the use of adjunctive supports, like the hospital, to protect the patient while the therapist engaged in expressive psychotherapy and maintained a neutral analytic stance.

Motivation for change.   There is a consensus in the field that expressive psychotherapy with any patient population, borderline or not, requires a substantial level of motivation to effect internal change. Simply seeking psychotherapy does not necessarily mean individuals are motivated to make changes in themselves; the wish may be to find an affirming or gratifying relationship. A related factor is the patient's perseverance, the ability and willingness to withstand an uncovering process that inevitably leads to psychic pain and discomfort.

Capacity to work in analytic space.   Ogden's (1986) concept of being able to create and maintain an analytic space, in which the dialectic between fantasy and reality is continually entertained, is another ego capacity that is necessary for expressive work. When patients become excessively fixated on the "reality" of their experience, for example, the analytic space is contracted or collapsed, and the exploration of the patient's inner world becomes drastically limited.

Impulse control/affective tolerance.   Patients who are ever on the verge of springing into thoughtless behavior make it virtually impossible to do exploratory work. Their penchant is to express feelings via action rather than through words, and hence the stress of uncovering unacceptable parts of the self would only exacerbate destructive and self-destructive behavior. These patients are usually the candidates for hospitalization, and when not hospitalized, their major need is a supportive treatment with an emphasis on directly enhancing and strengthening their behavioral controls.

Proneness to externalization. Patients who are given to project or externalize the source of their anxiety and conflicts are less amenable to exploring their inner worlds than patients who are given to looking inward for the source of their difficulties. Several writers have emphasized the difficulty, indeed the error, in attempting to use confrontive or interpretive techniques with those patients who are using paranoid-projective defenses. These patients require a relatively slow-moving, noninterpretive approach in which they are permitted to let go slowly of the projections at their own pace.

Psychological-mindedness. Expressive work requires that patients be capable of alternating between experiencing feelings and reflecting about them and between openly expressing themselves and observing the meanings and significance of their behavior. In some ways, psychological-mindedness is the result of possessing the other ego capacities to a sufficient degree: a low degree of narcissistic vulnerability, good control over impulses, and a tendency to internalize rather than externalize.

Relationship Factors

Narcissistic vulnerability. Practically all writers emphasized the importance of narcissistic vulnerability in modifying or curtailing expressive uncovering work. All borderline patients share a deficiency in self-esteem and a conviction that they are not valued or desired by others. Hence, self-understanding is the last item on the treatment agenda of many of these patients. Rather, they are intent on finding validation and affirmation as worthwhile and acceptable people. Some writers have emphasized the narcissistic rage that gets mobilized in the patients when their needs for affirmation are frustrated. The recent emphases on positivizing interventions or interpreting within the context of support are techniques intended to help the narcissistically vulnerable patient to listen to, to hear, and hopefully to accept the therapist's observations.

Mirroring or idealizing transferences. Kohut's (1977) characterization of these narcissistic transferences as requiring slow, nonintensive work is accepted by a number of writers on the borderline patient. Insofar as these patients are seen as needing the therapist to provide the empathic reparenting that they missed in their early development, an early interpretive approach is seen as counterproductive.

Distancing and counterdependency. Some writers have observed that patients whose preferred relationship mode is to distance themselves (seen in paranoid and schizoid individuals) present a more formidable obstacle to expressive work than those who are clinging and dependent. Interpretive work requires a sufficient degree of openness and willingness to share intimate details of one's life, and the distancing patient finds this task extremely threatening. The clinging patient, on the other hand, is usually more amenable to open expression of feelings.

Clinging and symbiotic needs. Although clinging symbiotic patients may be more able to communicate openly, they do not necessarily respond appreciatively to the therapist's interpretive efforts. On the contrary, some writers recognized that the clinging patient views therapeutic interpretations as unwelcome efforts by the therapist to encourage separation and distancing. Hence, the recommendation is to move slowly and carefully in interpreting symbiotic wishes.

Sadistic or erotized transference. Even those authors who have recommended a slow-moving method in dealing with borderline patients, for the most part postponing interpretive work until an adequate therapeutic alliance has been established, believe that extreme manifestations of erotized transference require immediate confrontation lest the patient be permitted to destroy or stalemate the treatment situation. Those interventions are viewed as risky prior to the development of an alliance but are regarded as preferable to the consequences of failing to attend to the patient's destructiveness. Extremely sadistic and hateful transferences that are designed to destroy the treatment also require immediate confrontation.

Flexibility Hypothesis

In addition to the developmental, ego, and relationship factors just described, we propose an additional major hypothesis that integrates some of the diverse ideas regarding a patient's closeness and distance propensities and their amenability to expressive work. Patients who manifest either behavioral extreme are not candidates for interpretation; those who alternate between the two extremes are more ready for uncovering work. Patients who maintain a close, symbiotic tie with their therapist indicate a weakness in selfobject differentiation and a need to use the treatment relationship to supply functions they are unable to fulfill on their own. Basically, such patients are seeking a symbiotic union with a maternal part-object, a merger with the good breast. They view the therapist as the soothing, magical protector from whom all good things derive. The conscious or unconscious compact they form in treatment is that they will be compliant, good children as long as the therapist will reciprocate with unending "supplies." Interpretations of their needs and unrealistic expectations may stress the separateness of patient and therapist and are likely to be experienced as a repetition of maternal failure and rejection.

Distant patients, on the other hand, are rigidly fixed in a defensive posture against seeking this symbiotic gratification. They have been described most clearly by Modell (1976) as encapsulated in a plastic bubble or glass jar; they feel constrained to remain affectively uncommunicative. Their hunger for a relationship is often indicated by seeking treatment, but their anxiety about the dangers of trusting themselves to others in a close setting makes it necessary to maintain a relatively impermeable barrier. Interpretations to these people involve an undue intrusion into their private domains, an effort to destroy their carefully protected islands of safety. Therapists who trespass this forbidden territory risk angry retaliation or a ruptured treatment. The two paradigms described here are presented in their most extreme form for heuristic purposes to convey the dimensions that must be considered in assessing a patient's readiness to use interpretations. Obviously, degrees of both closeness and distance must be considered.

The primary indicators of the borderline patient's amenability to interpretation are not only attenuated degrees of closeness-distance behavior but also manifestations of flexibility in their response patterns. If these patients alternate between the two behaviors, they are most likely to possess a greater readiness for accepting both the intimacy and the separateness involved in a transference interpretation (Horwitz 1985).

Therapists must attempt to differentiate between pathological and healthy alternation. At one extreme is the involuntary, automatic, poorly controlled alternation of ego states Kernberg (1976) described as characterizing many borderline patients. They oscillate between split self and object representations because of poorly integrated self and object internalizations. If these oscillations show little or no combination with their counterpart representations, and if the splitting is profound, the reactions are more pathognomonic and relatively unamenable to interpretation.

On the other hand, oscillations that have the earmarks of greater integration between good and bad internal representations are a positive sign. In these instances, the patient is likely to be communicating a readiness for the intimacy of transference exploration while retaining a necessary sense of separateness and autonomy. In other words, healthier, more adaptive alternation and regulation of closeness and distance is evident.

Summary

In this chapter, we focus on the issue of the optimal treatment strategy in the psychotherapy of borderline patients. More specifically, what kinds of borderline patients respond better to expressive methods, and which patients require a less intensive, more supportive approach? Our study assumed that the borderline diagnosis represents a continuum or spectrum ranging from high-level cases close to the neurotic border to low-level patients close to the psychotic border. The majority of writers have used a "lumping" strategy in which they proposed one general approach to the average, modal patient, while mentioning some exceptions for those persons who deviate from the majority. We believe that clearer diagnostic differentiations based on ego functions, relationship patterns, and developmental considerations will lead to the appropriate treatment approaches for a particular type of patient.

References

Abend SM, Porder MS, Willick MS: Borderline Patients: Psychoanalytic Perspectives. New York, International Universities Press, 1983

Adler G: The myth of the alliance with borderline patients. Am J Psychiatry 136:642–645, 1979

Adler G: Borderline Psychopathology and Its Treatment. New York, Jason Aronson, 1985

American Psychiatric Association: Diagnostic and Statistical Manual of Mental Disorders, 3rd Edition, Revised. Washington, DC, American Psychiatric Association, 1987

Andrulonis PA, Glueck BC, Stroebel CF, et al: Organic brain dysfunction and the borderline syndrome. Psychiatr Clin North Am 4:47–66, 1981

Boyer LB: Working with a borderline patient. Psychoanal Q 46:386–424, 1977

Brandchaft B, Stolorow RD: The borderline concept: an intersubjective viewpoint, in The Borderline Patient: Emerging Concepts in Diagnoses, Psychodynamics and Treatment, Vol 2. Edited by Grotstein JS, Solomon MF, Lang JA. Hillsdale, NJ, Analytic Press, 1987, pp 103–125

Buie DH, Adler G: Definitive treatment of the borderline patient. International Journal of Psychoanalysis and Psychotherapy 9:51–87, 1982/1983

Carpenter CJ, Gold JM, Fenton WS: Neuropsychological testing results in borderline inpatients. Paper presented at the 146th annual meeting of the American Psychiatric Association, San Francisco, CA, May 22–27, 1993

Chessick RD: Intensive Psychotherapy of the Borderline Patient. New York, Jason Aronson, 1977

Chessick RD: A practical approach to the psychotherapy of the borderline patient. Am J Psychother 33:531–546, 1979

Chessick RD: Intensive psychotherapy of a borderline patient. Arch Gen Psychiatry 39:413–419, 1982

Cornelius JR, Soloff PH, George AWA, et al: An evaluation of the significance of selected neuropsychiatric abnormalities in the etiology of borderline personality disorder. Journal of Personality Disorders 3:19–25, 1989

Epstein L: Countertransferences with borderline patients, in Countertransference: The Therapist's Contribution to the Therapeutic Situation. Edited by Epstein L, Feiner AH. New York, Jason Aronson, 1979, pp 375–405

Gabbard GO: Technical approaches to transference hate in the analysis of borderline patients. Int J Psychoanal 272:625–637, 1991

Gabbard GO, Wilkinson SM: Management of Countertransference With Borderline Patients. Washington, DC, American Psychiatric Press, 1994

Giovacchini PL: Treatment of Primitive Mental States. New York, Jason Aronson, 1979

Grinker RR, Werble B, Drye RC: The Borderline Syndrome: A Behavioral Study of Ego-Functions. New York, Basic Books, 1968

Gunderson JG: Borderline Personality Disorder. Washington, DC, American Psychiatric Press, 1984

Gunderson JG, Frank AF, Ronningstam EF, et al: Early discontinuance of borderline patients from psychotherapy. J Nerv Ment Dis 177:38–42, 1989

Horwitz L: Clinical Prediction in Psychotherapy. New York, Jason Aronson, 1974

Horwitz L: Divergent views on the treatment of borderline patients. Bull Menninger Clin 49:525–545, 1985

Hurt SW, Clarkin JF: Borderline personality disorder: prototypic typology and the development of treatment manuals. Psychiatric Annals 20:13–18, 1990

Judd PH, Ruff RM: Neuropsychological dysfunction in borderline personality disorder. Journal of Personality Disorders 7:275–284, 1993

Kernberg OF: Borderline Conditions and Pathological Narcissism. New York, Jason Aronson, 1975

Kernberg OF: Technical considerations in the treatment of borderline personality organization. J Am Psychoanal Assoc 24:795–829, 1976

Kernberg OF: Severe Personality Disorders: Psychotherapeutic Strategies. New Haven, CT, Yale University Press, 1984

Kernberg OF, Burstein ED, Coyne L, et al (eds): Psychotherapy and psychoanalysis: final report of the Menninger Foundation's Psychotherapy Research Project. Bull Menninger Clin 36:3–275, 1972

Kernberg OF, Selzer MA, Koenigsberg HW, et al: Psychodynamic Psychotherapy of Borderline Patients. New York, Basic Books, 1989

Klein M: Notes on some schizoid mechanisms (1946), in Envy and Gratitude and Other Works, 1946–1963. New York, Free Press, 1975, pp 1–24

Knight RP: Borderline states, in Psychoanalytic Psychiatry and Psychology: Clinical and Theoretical Papers, Vol 1. Edited by Knight RP, Friedman CR. New York, International Universities Press, 1954, pp 97–109

Kohut H: The Restoration of the Self. New York, International Universities Press, 1977

Kolb JE, Gunderson JG: Book review of *Psychodynamic Psychotherapy of Borderline Patients* by OF Kernberg et al. International Review of Psychoanalysis 17:513–516, 1990

Mahler MS, Pine F, Bergman A: The Psychological Birth of the Human Infant: Symbiosis and Individuation. New York, Basic Books, 1975

Malan DH: The Frontier of Brief Psychotherapy: An Example of the Convergence of Research and Clinical Practice. New York, Plenum, 1976

Masterson JF: Psychotherapy of the Borderline Adult: A Developmental Approach. New York, Brunner/Mazel, 1976

Meissner WW: Psychotherapy of the paranoid patient, in Technical Factors in the Treatment of the Severely Disturbed Patient. Edited by Giovacchini PL, Boyer LB. New York, Jason Aronson, 1982, pp 349–384

Meissner WW: The Borderline Spectrum: Differential Diagnosis and Developmental Issues. New York, Jason Aronson, 1984

Meissner WW: Treatment of Patients in the Borderline Spectrum. Northvale, NJ, Jason Aronson, 1988

Modell AH: The "holding environment" and the therapeutic action of psychoanalysis. J Am Psychoanal Assoc 24:285–307, 1976

Ogden TH: The Matrix of the Mind: Object Relations and the Psychoanalytic Dialogue. Northvale, NJ, Jason Aronson, 1986

O'Leary KM, Cowdry RW: Neuropsychological testing results in borderline personality disorder, in Biological and Neurobehavioral Studies of Borderline Personality Disorder. Edited by Silk KR. Washington, DC, American Psychiatric Press, 1994, pp 127–157

O'Leary KM, Brouwers P, Gardner DL, et al: Neuropsychological testing of patients with borderline personality disorder. Am J Psychiatry 148:106–111, 1991

Pine F: The interpretive moment: variations on classical themes. Bull Menninger Clin 48:54–71, 1984

Piper WE, Azim HFA, Joyce AS, et al: Transference interpretations, therapeutic alliance, and outcome in short-term individual psychotherapy. Arch Gen Psychiatry 48:946–953, 1991

Schaffer ND: The borderline patient and affirmative interpretation. Bull Menninger Clin 50:148–162, 1986

Skodol AE, Buckley P, Charles E: Is there a characteristic pattern to the treatment history of clinic outpatients with borderline personality? J Nerv Ment Dis 171:405–410, 1983

Stevenson J, Meares R: An outcome study of psychotherapy for patients with borderline personality disorder. Am J Psychiatry 149:358–362, 1992

Stone MH: The Fade of Borderline Patients: Successful Outcome and Psychiatric Practice. New York, Guilford, 1990

Strupp HH, Binder JL: Psychotherapy in a New Key: A Guide to Time-Limited Dynamic Psychotherapy. New York, Basic Books, 1984

Volkan VD: Six Steps in the Treatment of Borderline Personality Organization. New York, Jason Aronson, 1987

Waldinger RJ: Intensive psychodynamic therapy with borderline patients: an overview. Am J Psychiatry 144:267–274, 1987

Waldinger RJ, Gunderson JG: Completed psychotherapies with borderline patients. Am J Psychother 38:190–202, 1984

Waldinger RJ, Gunderson JG: Effective Psychotherapy With Borderline Patients: Case Studies. Washington, DC, American Psychiatric Press, 1987

Wallerstein RS: Forty-Two Lives in Treatment: A Study of Psychoanalysis and Psychotherapy. New York, Guilford, 1986

Yeomans FE, Gutfreund J, Selzer MA, et al: Factors related to dropouts by borderline patients: treatment contract and therapeutic alliance. Journal of Psychotherapy Practice and Research 3:16–24, 1994

Zetzel ER: A developmental approach to the borderline patient. Am J Psychiatry 127:867–871, 1971

Effect of Interventions
on the
Therapeutic Alliance

Although stirring controversy within analytic circles as a whole, the concept of therapeutic alliance is recognized almost universally as a critical variable in the treatment of borderline patients. Almost every writer emphasizes that the difficulty of engaging typical borderline patients in treatment, and helping them to remain in treatment, is compounded by the impaired quality of object relations of this population. Typically, these patients have experienced severe disappointments and frustrations at the hands of significant people and therefore, to a greater or lesser degree, have a built-in wariness of all relationships. Furthermore, they react to the inevitable misunderstandings and empathic failures that occur in relationships with intense feelings of injury and outrage, usually leading to a disruption of the connection.

A Key Concept in the
Treatment of Borderline Disorders

Meissner (1988) viewed the formation of a therapeutic alliance as crucial to establishing an effective psychotherapeutic process with borderline patients. He endorsed the definition given by Gutheil and Havens (1979) as "the therapeutic split in the ego which allows the analyst to work with the healthier elements in the patient against resistance and pathology" (p. 479). In operationalizing this definition, Meissner included several elements that contribute to establishing a viable therapeutic alliance: contractual arrangements regarding fees, payment, appointments, and confidentiality; the mutually agreed on goals for the psychotherapy; and a contractual understanding regarding the roles and responsibilities of each party. Meissner suggested that the therapeutic alliance involves certain aspects of the therapist-patient relationship that are not subsumed by transference or by the real relationship. He also stressed that the therapeutic alliance is not a concept that is confined to the patient but rather involves contributions from both therapist and patient. He specifically noted that the therapist's attitude of expecting meaningful involvement in the process by the patient is a key element in establishing a therapeutic alliance.

In Meissner's (1988) view, the outcome of psychotherapy is substantially influenced by the nature of the therapeutic alliance formed by patient and therapist. He also pointed out, however, that the patient's capacity to maintain a therapeutic split in the ego varies considerably along the borderline spectrum. At the higher level of the spectrum, one sees subtle erosions; dramatic disruptions are more characteristic of lower-level borderline patients. In outlining his technique, Meissner stressed the need to invest a good deal of effort into repairing alliance disruptions throughout the course of treatment.

Writers who espouse quite different views regarding the optimal treatment of borderline patients seem to agree that an important objective of treatment is to strengthen the alliance. Chessick (1979) believed that the therapist's first task is to develop and strengthen the alliance. Masterson (1976) similarly suggested that the first phase of treatment, which may last for months or even years, must be devoted to helping patients overcome their initial resistances to establishing a therapeutic alliance in which they begin to rely on the relationship for help in overcoming their symptoms and self-destructive behavior. Meissner (1988) also stated that the major problem in the therapy of borderline patients is initiating, strengthening, and developing the therapeutic alliance. He suggested that creating a therapeutic alliance with borderline patients is demanding and makes the real personality of the therapist more crucial than would be true with neurotic patients. This observation was consonant with the findings of the Menninger Psychotherapy Research Project (Horwitz 1974). Kernberg (1976) also regarded the alliance as an essential component of treatment. When transference intensity threatens to overwhelm the alliance, and the observing ego of the borderline patient becomes compromised, the therapist may have to take active measures to strengthen the alliance. The real relationship with the therapist is potentially therapeutic per se and may constitute an important reparative emotional experience in the treatment.

Although recognizing the crucial importance of the relationship in the therapeutic process with borderline patients, Adler (1979) took issue with the prevailing notion of the alliance as applied to these patients. Referring to the "fallacy" of applying the concept to this population, Adler contended that the capacity for an alliance is confined to those higher level, neurotic patients who are capable of maintaining firm boundaries and differentiating between the self and objects. The close, gratifying relationship between borderline patients and their therapists, according to Adler, is a function of the soothing and nurturing effect of the relatively undifferentiated self-object transferences and should not be confused with the more mature, realistic therapeutic alliance. In the course of a successful treatment, the reliable and helpful behavior of the therapist gradually becomes internalized and structuralized, permitting the patient eventually to be able to develop a true alliance. Although Adler's cautions regarding the levels and maturity of positive relationships are well taken, we believe that the alliance may include a broad range of developmental levels and that it is always rooted to some degree in archaic and primitive transferences.

Most researchers agree that the positive relationship that develops between borderline patients and their therapists, particularly as related to real rather than idealized aspects of the relationship, plays a significant role in the curative process. A major finding of the Menninger Psychotherapy Research Project was that supportive psychotherapy, in which interpreting and uncovering unconscious conflict were minimal and which largely rode on a positive dependent transference, was not only effective but also contributed to stable structural change (Horwitz 1974; Wallerstein 1986). One explanation proposed for this finding was that the patients successfully internalized the therapeutic alliance and thus achieved a stable generalization of the benevolent aspects of their relationship to the therapist (Horwitz 1974).

The Therapeutic Alliance Controversy

Even though the analytic theories of borderline treatment have relied heavily on the concept of therapeutic alliance, some psychoanalysts have been quite critical of the validity of the concept. Two factors enter into their criticisms, one of which is clearly based on a confusion of the alliance with treatment prescriptions. The background to this development was the pioneering article by Zetzel (1956) in which she wedded certain technical recommendations with the efforts to enhance patient collaboration. The context of her contribution was the effort to broaden the scope of psychoanalysis to include the treatment of narcissistic and borderline conditions. Specifically, she suggested that the analyst should not be too silent for too long without making supportive comments that acknowledge the patient's distress, anxiety, and fear. Hence, for some analytic authors (Brenner 1979; Curtis 1979; Kanzer 1975), focus on the alliance came to imply supportive, nonanalytic therapeutic strategies. Although supportive measures may sometimes be used to enhance the alliance, this connection does not occur universally or unvaryingly. Greenson (1967), another important contributor in this area, strongly held to the view that a major vehicle in strengthening the alliance, particularly with regard to specific areas of difficulty for the patient, was to interpret the patient's resistances.

The second criticism of the concept is based on the view that the alliance may be reduced to a variety of transferences (Brenner 1979). This point of view has been critiqued by Frieswyk et al. (1984), and the highlights of their review follow. Greenson (1967) defined the alliance as "the relatively nonneurotic rational relationship between patient and analyst which makes it possible for the patient to work purposefully in the analytic situation" (p. 46). This relatively neutralized relationship makes possible the patient's cooperation with the analyst. The distinction between the alliance and the transference is not an absolute one, and in fact, the alliance is influenced by a core of object-relations capacities that are essential to forming a trusting relationship. Freud (1912/1958) originally described this as the "unobjectionable positive transference"; Greenacre (1968) referred to these positive feelings as "primary transference"; Stone (1961) used "primordial transference"; and Langs (1976) referred to the "matrix transference." All are associated with an underlying hope that the treatment will result in positive change and often contain magic and unrealistically tinged omnipotent wishes. Also included are elements of the infantile neurosis that, according to Greenson (1967), contribute to the alliance and eventually require analysis. Furthermore, the activation of certain transferences may temporarily obscure the alliance so that the patient is no longer able to work realistically in the relationship.

However, separating this relatively conflict-free aspect of the relationship from those components that are neurotically determined is useful. The alliance concept emphasizes the intactness of the realistic perceptions of patients and their capacity to retain an observing ego, thus enabling them to engage in constructive and collaborative analytic work. In other words, despite transference determinants to the alliance and perhaps temporary intrusion and interference, keeping these two aspects of the therapeutic relationship separately defined has heuristic value.

Alliance as Patient Collaboration

The therapeutic alliance is typically defined as an interactional variable in which both the patient and the therapist make significant contributions (Meissner 1988). Although this view of the alliance is self-evident, our research group was impressed by the common clinical observation that difficulties with the therapeutic alliance as described in clinical presentations are almost always discussed in terms of the patient's characteristics. Researchers have generally recognized that the patient is the one who sets the limit on the kind of relationship that can be established, even though the therapist's contribution may be quite significant. This observation tends to be confirmed by the research finding (Hartley 1985) that the patient's perceptions and contributions to the alliance, rather than the therapist's behaviors, best predict successful outcome. These observations led our research group to focus specifically on the patient's collaboration with the therapist as the marker variable and final common pathway of the patient's alliance (Colson et al. 1988).

This formulation does not minimize or slight the contribution of the therapist to the therapeutic process nor to the alliance. Rather, it encourages a clearer delineation between the contributions of patient and therapist to their joint effort. By separating the two components, therapists are in a better position to evaluate the extent to which they contribute to the patient's collaborative efforts.

Also, we were influenced by the fact that collaboration is a behavioral variable, as opposed to an attitudinal one encompassing trust, optimism, and other internal experiences. Our view was that all the factors contributing to the alliance, including the patient's characterological attitudes, as well as the therapist's personal qualities and professional skills, will contribute to the final common pathway of the patient's ability to collaborate. Collaboration would then be assessed by the constructiveness of the patient's work in a session, including the ability to bring significant issues into the treatment and the ability to make use of the therapist's contribution.

Shifts in the Collaboration as Mini-Outcomes

Greenberg (1991) observed that psychotherapy research is undergoing a paradigm shift from attempting to prove the efficacy of psychotherapy to a focus on discovering the processes that contribute to change. Our study is one example of this evolutionary shift insofar as it engages in a microanalysis of events within a psychotherapy session. If we were interested in comparing the general efficacy of supportive versus expressive interventions with borderline patients, we would have designed a group comparison study or clinical trial of matched groups of borderline patients receiving two different modalities. But we were interested in learning more about the immediate fate of various types of interventions in the therapy hours. Accordingly, we opted to do an intensive study of individual cases in which the effect of particular kinds of interventions on certain types of patients is examined with as much objectivity as possible.

An underlying assumption of this work is that accurate, empathic, and timely interventions by the therapist will result in positive shifts in collaboration, usually within the same session. Whether the intervention is supportive or expressive, an interpretation or a sound piece of advice, whether a confrontation or a simple request to elaborate—the intervention that best fits the needs of the patient at that moment is what will tend to induce these patients to increase their efforts to work more closely with the therapist to receive maximum benefits from the process. Conversely, a failure in empathy, a poorly timed interpretation, or a failure to offer much-needed support may result in a downward shift in the alliance and in the patient's collaboration.

These shifts represent mini-outcomes in the sense that the cumulative effect of repeated shifts in either a positive or negative direction will gradually lead to an overall outcome that is either positive or negative. The method of detecting within-session shifts allows us to answer the main question we posed at the outset of the study: What kinds of interventions are best suited for what kinds of patients? Positive shifts in the alliance are not only indicators of the suitability of the intervention, but are positive mini-outcomes that ultimately may be aggregated to lead to a favorable overall outcome.

Research Strategy

Overview

In this chapter. we describe a collaborative study by six senior clinicians at The Menninger Clinic, all of whom were experienced in the theory and practice of psychoanalytic psychotherapy. This intensive study focused on three cases in which the psychotherapy process and interaction between patient and therapist were investigated in minute detail. We audiotaped all the psychotherapy sessions and worked from typed transcripts of randomly selected psychotherapy hours. More details are available in Appendix B.

In our study of the issue of the use of supportive versus expressive therapeutic strategies, we adopted one major assumption. We agreed with those writers who took the view of a borderline continuum or spectrum, ranging from patients close to the neurotic line to those close to a psychotic condition, comprising a wide variety of character types. Our guiding view was that this variation should dictate treatment strategies. We decided that our focus would be on determining which kind of borderline patient responds best to a predominantly expressive approach and which does better with a mainly supportive treatment.

We assessed two major classes of variables—those relating to the kinds of interventions used by the therapist, ranging from supportive to expressive, and those relating to the therapeutic alliance, which we operationalized as the patient's ability to collaborate with the therapist. We regarded the therapeutic interventions as our independent variable, the varying input provided by the therapist that in turn influenced the dependent variable, the therapeutic alliance, marked by the patient's ability to collaborate at any given time.

Our principal objective was to assess the optimal balance of expressive and supportive interventions for different types of borderline patients. We employed two time perspectives—longitudinal (over the entire course of treatment) and cross-sectional (samples of selected sessions)—to generate running profiles of therapist interventions. In doing so, we examined how the therapist's comments interacted with the patient's characteristics and how both patient characteristics and therapist interventions related to the outcome of the therapy. We also studied the possible links between within-session shifts in the patient's collaboration and the therapist's prior interventions within the session, keeping in mind that a patient's reactions within a given session may also be related to long-range effects and to the quality of the therapeutic relationship.

A subgroup of three clinician-judges assessed the therapist's interventions and selected one of seven types of intervention categories to describe each of the therapist's statements. Categories ranged from the most expressive to the most supportive (i.e., interpretation, confrontation, clarification, encouragement to elaborate, empathy, advice/encouragement, and affirmation). In addition, each intervention was classified as either a transference or extratransference comment. The judges rated the adequacy of each intervention based on its accuracy, tact, timing, and appropriateness and made a global rating of therapist competency. Finally, since we were focusing on the issue of supportiveness and expressiveness, the judges rated each overall session with a score on these two dimensions.

A separate subgroup of three clinician-judges assessed a key facet of the therapeutic alliance, namely, the patient's collaboration with the therapist. We were primarily interested in the ability of the patient to bring in significant content and to make productive use of the therapist's contributions. The judges were primarily interested in detecting upward or downward shifts in the patient's collaboration, whenever they occurred in a session. We were especially interested in determining whether the shifts were related to the therapist's interventions. In addition, the judges made overall ratings of collaboration for each session, and we rated the widely known Luborsky Working Alliance Scales (Luborsky 1976).

The ratings for the various patient collaboration measures and for the therapist interventions measures were made by two separate subgroups of three clinicians each. All clinicians first worked independently and then met with their subgroup to form consensus decisions. Later, both subgroups met as an entire research team to use their best clinical judgment in determining a possible linkage between the upward or downward shifts in collaboration and the preceding interventions by the therapist (see Appendix D, Table D–3, Table D–7, and Table D–11). Once again, each of the six clinicians worked independently and then the team reached a consensus. Sometimes the shift was deemed unrelated to the therapist's contributions, sometimes a series of interventions were thought to be contributory, and at other times one particular statement by the therapist was viewed as crucial in determining the shift in collaboration.

Two additional pairs of clinician-judges, not otherwise associated with the main research group, made some further judgments. The prediction subgroup was given the initial clinical evaluation and asked to make judgments regarding the extent to which expressive and/or supportive measures would be used by the therapist to deal with particular conflicts or problems. This subgroup also rated the patients with regard to their pattern of closeness and distance as a way of helping to assess the flexibility hypothesis. The outcome subgroup examined materials both from the initial assessment of the patient and from the outcome and follow-up period and assessed the changes the patient had achieved in psychotherapy (see Appendix D, Table D–1, Table D–5, and Table D–9). Once again, the judgments by the two clinicians on each team were first done independently, followed by a discussion to reach a consensus.

Intensive Study of Single Cases

At the outset of our study in the early 1980s, the investigators shared the conviction that progress in learning more about optimal techniques of psychotherapy required careful study of recorded sessions. The design of such studies should consist of an intensive study of single cases as described by Chassen (1979), Barlow and Hersen (1984), and Rice and Greenberg (1984). We agree with these authors that group comparison and correlational studies are most appropriate in a fairly advanced stage of psychotherapy research after hypotheses have been explored and measuring instruments have been tested using individualized intensive methods. There was a growing conviction among psychotherapy researchers that group comparison studies had insufficiently identified major factors in the therapeutic change process (Waskow 1984). To achieve a better understanding of how moment-to-moment changes come about, we decided to use a strategy of discovery that assessed therapeutic change microscopically. Since that early stage of our thinking, Abend et al. (1983) used a single-case methodology focusing on detailed process notes to study a psychoanalytic approach to borderline psychopathology. In addition, Waldinger and Gunderson (1987) reported a study of five borderline patients in extended psychoanalytic psychotherapy.

Our study is not a series of clinical case studies with the typical anecdotal method. Rather, we embarked on an exploratory study using samples of recorded treatment hours that we examined with empirically derived rating instruments. The detailed study of single cases allows us to supplement systematic ratings of relevant variables with qualitative observations of events, other than those measured, that may influence the psychotherapy process.

We recognize that the single-case method inevitably must cope with the problem of generalizability. We were fortunate in our selection of cases that our patients spanned a broad portion of the borderline spectrum: one was clearly a high-level borderline patient, one clearly was at the midlevel, and the third was somewhere between those two poles. Also, to what extent may we claim that the findings regarding a particular case is applicable to other similar cases? Obviously, single-case researchers and their collaborators need continually to add more patients to their universe to correct and refine their hypotheses. Our hope is that this study will stimulate others to use similar methods.

Patients

Our initial selection criteria for the three patients included in this study were that they must be 18 years of age, in psychotherapy at least twice a week for most of their treatment, and of at least average intelligence. The patients were drawn from those psychotherapies begun by members of the research team at approximately the time the study was initiated. The patients must have had a primary diagnosis of borderline personality disorder, as defined by DSM-III-R (American Psychiatric Association 1987), determined by the usual intake diagnostic procedures of The Menninger Clinic, which include a psychiatric case study, a social history, and comprehensive psychological testing. On the basis of the clinical material, each member of the research team independently evaluated each patient on the presence or absence of each of the DSM-III-R criteria for borderline personality disorder to ensure each patient met at least minimum criteria for the diagnosis. In addition, members of the research team conducted an initial research assessment using the Diagnostic Interview for Borderline Patients (DIB) (Gunderson et al. 1981) and reached a team consensus score on this scale.

The three patients selected for the study included two women and one man. Two of those were in a psychiatric hospital and partial hospitalization services for some portion of their psychotherapy, and all three received psychotropic medication at some point during the psychotherapy process.

Research Team Composition

The core research team consisted of six senior psychotherapists at The Menninger Clinic, four of whom had psychoanalytic training.

Each member of the research team had extensive experience in conducting psychoanalytic psychotherapy with borderline patients. Three members of the research team were able to find suitable cases and volunteered to tape record them for purposes of the research.

The six-member research team divided into two three-member subgroups. One subgroup assessed patient collaboration, and the other subgroup assessed therapist interventions. The composition of the subgroups remained the same throughout the research project. Dividing the research team into two subgroups ensured that the ratings of patient collaboration and therapist interventions would be independent.

In addition to the six-member research team, two pairs of clinician-raters assisted in the research. One of these pairs, the prediction raters, made predictions about the optimal therapeutic strategy for each of the three patients, based on the initial clinical material for each case. The prediction raters were two highly experienced clinicians, one a psychoanalyst and the other an experienced psychodynamically oriented psychotherapist. The other pair of additional raters, the outcome raters, assessed each patient's functioning at the beginning of psychotherapy and at follow-up to determine the nature and extent of change. The outcome raters were also highly experienced clinicians and psychotherapists, one a psychoanalyst.

These additional raters, the prediction and outcome pairs, were employed to provide independent assessment of the optimal therapeutic strategy and the treatment outcome. Unlike the research team members, they had no knowledge of the extended psychotherapy process.

References

Abend SM, Porder MS, Willick MS: Borderline Patients: Psychoanalytic Perspectives. New York, International Universities Press, 1983

Adler G: The myth of the alliance with borderline patients. Am J Psychiatry 136:642–645, 1979

American Psychiatric Association: Diagnostic and Statistical Manual of Mental Disorders, 3rd Edition, Revised. Washington, DC, American Psychiatric Association, 1987

Barlow DH, Hersen M: Single Case Experimental Designs: Strategies for Studying Behavior Change. New York, Pergamon, 1984

Brenner C: Working alliance, therapeutic alliance, and transference. J Am Psychoanal Assoc 27 (suppl):137–157, 1979

Chassen JB: Research Design in Clinical Psychology and Psychiatry, 2nd Edition. New York, Wiley, 1979

Chessick RD: A practical approach to the psychotherapy of the borderline patient. Am J Psychother 33:531–546, 1979

Colson DB, Horwitz L, Allen JG, et al: Patient collaboration as a criterion for the therapeutic alliance. Psychoanalytic Psychology 5:259–268, 1988

Curtis HC: The concept of therapeutic alliance: implications for the "widening scope." J Am Psychoanal Assoc 27 (suppl):159–192, 1979

Freud S: The dynamics of transference (1912), in The Standard Edition of the Complete Psychological Works of Sigmund Freud, Vol 12. Translated and edited by Strachey J. London, Hogarth Press, 1958, pp 97–108

Frieswyk SH, Colson DB, Allen JG: Conceptualizing the therapeutic alliance from a psychoanalytic perspective. Psychotherapy 21:460–464, 1984

Greenacre P: The psychoanalytic process, transference, and acting out. Int J Psychoanal 49:211–218, 1968

Greenberg LS: Research on the process of change. Psychotherapy Research 1:3–16, 1991

Greenson RR: The Technique and Practice of Psychoanalysis, Vol 1. New York, International Universities Press, 1967

Gunderson JG, Kolb JE, Austin V: The Diagnostic Interview for Borderline Patients. Am J Psychiatry 138:896–903, 1981

Gutheil TH, Havens LL: The therapeutic alliance: contemporary meanings and confusions. International Review of Psychoanalysis 6:467–481, 1979

Hartley DE: Research on the therapeutic alliance in psychotherapy, in Psychiatry Update: American Psychiatric Association Annual Review, Vol 4. Edited by Hales RE, Frances AJ. Washington, DC, American Psychiatric Press, 1985, pp 532–549

Horwitz L: Clinical Prediction in Psychotherapy. New York, Jason Aronson, 1974

Kanzer M: The therapeutic and working alliances. International Journal of Psychoanalysis and Psychotherapy 4:48–68, 1975

Kernberg OF: Technical considerations in the treatment of borderline personality organization. J Am Psychoanal Assoc 24:795–829, 1976

Langs R: The Therapeutic Interaction, Vol 2: A Critical Overview and Synthesis. New York, Jason Aronson, 1976

Luborsky L: Helping alliances in psychotherapy, in Successful Psychotherapy. Edited by Claghorn J. New York, Brunner/Mazel, 1976, pp 92–116

Masterson JF: Psychotherapy of the Borderline Adult: A Developmental Approach. New York, Brunner/Mazel, 1976

Meissner WW: Treatment of Patients in the Borderline Spectrum. Northvale, NJ, Jason Aronson, 1988

Rice LH, Greenberg L (eds): Patterns of Change. New York, Guilford, 1984

Stone L: The Psychoanalytic Situation: An Examination of Its Developmental and Essential Nature. New York, International Universities Press, 1961

Waldinger RJ, Gunderson JG: Effective Psychotherapy With Borderline Patients: Case Studies. Washington, DC, American Psychiatric Press, 1987

Wallerstein RS: Forty-Two Lives in Treatment: A Study of Psychoanalysis and Psychotherapy. New York, Guilford, 1986

Waskow IE: New directions in NIMH psychotherapy research programs. Paper presented to Society for Psychotherapy Research, Lake Louise, Ontario, Canada, June 1984

Zetzel ER: Current concepts of transference. Int J Psychoanal 37:369–376, 1956

CHAPTER 3

Mr. Black

At the start of psychotherapy, Mr. Black[1] was a high school teacher in his mid-30s, recently separated from his wife and two children, who had moved to a distant city. At the time the patient began psychotherapy, he was hospitalized and being treated with antidepressant medication. He had been hospitalized for the previous 5 months because of a serious depression accompanied by suicidal thoughts. His decompensation was preceded by a number of serious losses: his father had died rather suddenly 1 year earlier; his wife had decided to separate and proceed with a divorce, largely because he had declared himself to be homosexual; and a troubled relationship with his principal made it unlikely that he could continue in his teaching position. Indeed, his intention to "come out of the closet" and openly declare himself a homosexual was forcing him to rethink his vocational future. The patient's own complaints were a negative self-image and serious concerns about suicide.

A highly intelligent and verbally facile man with a particular talent in the arts, Mr. Black was constantly plagued by his conviction that he was unacceptable to other people unless he complied with their expectations and gratified their needs. He developed an as-if person-

---

[1] Preliminary data on this same patient were reported in a previous communication (Gabbard et al. 1988).

ality in which a pleasant, agreeable, and compliant self was a facade hiding feelings of weakness, stupidity, and self-despised homosexuality. Paradoxically, he also nurtured feelings of grandiosity about his talents and his ability to manipulate others, and he occasionally permitted himself to believe concretely and magically that God was guiding his future, an idea closely approaching a Christ-like fantasy. Nevertheless, he was filled with rage that God, as well as other important figures in his life, were not to be trusted and would eventually disappoint him. He constantly sought approval by his superiors, but underneath he was resentful and rebellious that others expected him to accommodate to their needs and wishes.

His sexual preference was for males as far back as he could remember. Embarrassed and despising himself for these urges, he sought to overcome them by marriage, only to discover some 8 years and two children later that he could no longer maintain a heterosexual facade, at which point he began having episodic homosexual contacts. Also disturbing him was that his pedophiliac fantasies were beginning to come dangerously close to overt expression.

An extensive battery of psychological tests was administered at the time of admission. The testing revealed a man overwhelmed by dysphoric affect. The quality of his depression was of someone "being attacked by ruthlessly sadistic internal persecutors intent on rubbing his nose in the excrement of his supposed perversions, weaknesses, and totally despicable self." The tormentors seemed to reflect primitive superego precursors, which had never been tamed into a reasonable semblance of a conscience. His ability to think clearly was compromised by the intensity of the affective forces within him. Distortions in his thinking were not of psychotic proportions, but serious reality aberrations were in evidence on psychological testing. Mr. Black seemed to experience himself as a patchwork combination of masculine and feminine, strong and weak, and good and evil. His experience of strength and masculinity was quickly associated with sadistic domination, exploitativeness, and unmanageable aggression. Strength was typically perceived as evil and was feared. He was gallantly attempting to hold on to a view of others as benign and potentially helpful, but he was losing ground in his ability to ward off fears and suspicions of others.

Both the psychiatric evaluation and the psychological testing pointed to a diagnosis of borderline personality organization, given his intense raw affective experiences that tended to disorganize his thinking, severe identity diffusion with a tendency toward polymorphous perverse sexuality, a split of both external and internal objects into all good or all bad, the primitive and unintegrated quality of his superego nuclei, and the generalized weakness of his overall defensive strategies. The psychologist predicted that further blows to his self-esteem could easily result in psychosis and serious suicidal behavior, which could grow out of a delusional sense that he needed to kill himself to appease his internal attackers.

The diagnosis of borderline personality disorder was further substantiated by the ratings of the research group using the DSM-III-R (American Psychiatric Association 1987) criteria. They first made independent ratings. Then they met to reach a consensus and found that the patient fulfilled five of the diagnostic criteria. A videotaped Gunderson et al. (1981) Diagnostic Interview for Borderline Patients (DIB) was also done, and a similar procedure was followed in which independent ratings were first made, followed by a consensus rating of 5, which did not fulfill Gunderson's criteria of 7 for the borderline diagnosis.

In formulating the nature of his illness, a prominent factor was a disturbed, unstable family in his early years. The patient's mother was an embittered, burdened woman, contemptuous of men and preoccupied with her own needs and interests. The father was somewhat approachable but often away from home trying to eke out a living. He was remembered as erratic and moody and given to temper outbursts, at which times the patient recalls being beaten with a razor strap. The middle of three children, the patient felt that his father favored his older sister and that his mother favored his younger brother, and he saw himself as the neglected outsider. Feeling insecurely bonded and tenuously loved by both his mother and father, he struggled mightily to find ways to please them and their surrogates by his achievements, his compliance, and his flattery. All the while he felt enraged at being found unacceptable for himself, and he nurtured a secret fantasy life in which he was powerful, loved, and, in particular, not dependent on unreliable parental figures. His struggle with sexuality was compounded by his mother's open abhorrence of males as beasts.

Predictions

Because the focus of this study is on the issue of supportive versus expressive interventions, we asked two clinician-judges who had no information about the treatment course to make an assessment of the patient by using the initial data and then to predict the optimal treatment strategy. These predictions are akin to the unspoken mental processes used by all clinicians because therapeutic interventions always involve implicit predictions regarding the patient's needs. The following is a summary of their consensus judgments.

The judges clearly opted for a mainly expressive treatment addressing the major issues the patient was likely to present. They anticipated much work to be done on his self-destructiveness associated with a "savage superego," hypomanic denial, and intermittent impulsivity. Next, they expected considerable work on his narcissistic vulnerability, his "patchwork self," his need to conceal his true self with an as-if veneer, and his alternating idealization-devaluation. They forecasted considerable emphasis on his regressive, acting-out tendencies, especially in relation to loss and separation. Finally, much work was likely to be done on the multiple losses he had experienced, particularly during the 2–3 years preceding the treatment. These were the issues that would require a predominantly expressive, uncovering approach, hopefully leading to insight and structural change.

On the other hand, they expected that certain kinds of structuring, reality confrontation, and advice might be necessary to help the patient control his tendencies toward impulsive, ill-advised, and self-destructive behavior. Also, they believed that his narcissistic vulnerability would not only require interpretation, but he would sometimes need more direct gratification via praise and empathic attunement for "quick self-esteem boosts" and management of depression.

Their predictions and recommendations were based on the following considerations:

■ A moderate-to-high degree of motivation to explore his conflicts that produced painful depressive reactions, despite a countervalent tendency to back away from affect-laden material, was evident. He seemed motivated to look beyond the veil of denial in many areas.

■ He possessed a high degree of intelligence and readiness to use this capacity in the service of understanding his inner life and conflicts.

■ He had an abiding need to experience empathic attunement with a parental figure that would permit him to share his hidden, true self and to give up his ungratifying as-if facade. His wish to become a more integrated, whole person in treatment spoke to a strategy of uncovering hidden parts of the self.

Course of Therapy

Mr. Black was in psychotherapy for 7 years. Consistent with the judges' predictions, the psychotherapy was predominantly expressive. Most of this period was at a frequency of three times per week, but in the fifth year appointments were tapered down to two times per week, and in the last year, to one session per week. He was seen for a total of 734 hours. He remained in the hospital for the first year and a half of the psychotherapy, largely because of his continuing suicidal ideation. On discharge he entered the partial hospitalization program, the intensity of which he decreased after the first several months, but he did not completely give it up until another 2 years had elapsed. Antidepressant medication continued throughout the period of his full and partial hospitalization.

The major impulse-defense configurations were uncovered, in particular his wish to be loved and nurtured countered by the conviction that he will be disappointed, hence his need to provide such gratification to himself. This conflict between wish and fear had become amply evident, both in his outside life and within the treatment relationship, and a long process of working through was necessary to help him modify an embedded character pattern.

The beginning phase of treatment was characterized by his effort to avoid becoming engaged with the therapist. He used his high intelligence and excellent verbal facility to keep the therapist from getting to know and understand him by delivering long-winded, obsessional monologues that were smoke screens in the service of affective noncommunication. He resembled Modell's (1976) description of the narcissistic patient who strives for self-sufficiency by enclosing himself within a cocoon, a plastic bubble, or a bell jar. Such sessions produced perplexity, irritation, and sleepiness in the therapist, and the patient required persistent prodding and confrontations. His early idealizations of the treater as a "super therapist" were intended to lull the therapist into a passive stance and provide him with a smug sense of self-satisfaction that would not disturb the patient's distance taking. He had a conscious fear of discovering that the therapist could actually become helpful to him, that he might become attached to the therapist, and that his self-sufficient stance would crumble. If that happened, he would be opening himself to inevitable frustration, disappointment, and eventually rage. Very early he began showing the pattern of taking his vacations at times different from the therapist, always with a good reason why this arrangement was necessary.

Paradoxically, Mr. Black began requesting with some persistence that the frequency of treatment be increased from three to four times a week. This request started early in treatment and periodically resurfaced, particularly in the context of interruptions. He contended that he did not have sufficient time to deal with all the issues he needed to discuss, and always in the background was the fact that his very generous insurance program would pay the increased cost. Also, consistent with his as-if orientation, he saw himself as having to talk mainly about what the therapist was interested in and believed that a fourth hour would give him the opportunity to talk about what *he* wanted to discuss. The therapist interpreted, rather than gratified, the patient's request, depending on the context in which it arose. In general, the therapist viewed the wish as an effort to test his interest and commitment to the relationship, and, particularly around times of interruptions such as vacations, Mr. Black wanted the therapist to counteract the conviction that he was eager to be rid of the patient. Toward the end of treatment, Mr. Black said that he never really accepted those interpretations, but he was aware of *wanting* to see the therapist as less invested in the relationship than he was, a fact that gave him a sense of moral superiority.

The predictors' expectation that the patient's harsh superego would be explored and uncovered in considerable detail was indeed the case. His strongly ingrained pattern of trying to discern what the therapist expected from him, his as-if personality, was accompanied by the patient's feeling masochistically exploited, deprived, and criticized. He quickly discovered that the therapist was interested in working with the transference, and he was constantly trying to anticipate when the therapist would be bringing it in, but he frequently complained that the therapist's interest prevented him from discussing essential issues going on outside the treatment relationship. He saw the therapist as attempting to make him give up the few pleasures he enjoyed in life and often tried to pull the therapist out of his position of therapeutic neutrality into revealing what he really thought about the patient and his behaviors. Mr. Black believed that the therapist was critical of him for his obesity and addiction to chocolates, for his homosexuality, and for his masturbation rituals. He thought the therapist would like to deprive him of these pleasures because of the sadistic enjoyment the therapist would derive from inflicting punishment on him.

In the very first session, Mr. Black wanted assurances that the therapist would not attempt to take away his homosexuality. Despite his efforts earlier in life to make a heterosexual adjustment, he viewed himself as a lifelong homosexual. His masturbation fantasies had been primarily about males, and in the entire period of treatment there was no inkling of heterosexual interest. He explicitly stated that his goal was to find a satisfactory homosexual marriage. There was little doubt in the therapist's mind that the patient's sexual orientation was deeply embedded in his character and probably had a genetic basis. In the first phase of treatment, the patient engaged in a flurry of transient affairs, was occasionally promiscuous, and cruised homosexual meeting places. For several years he consistently avoided a stable sexual relationship with the possible exception of one individual, a much younger man, someone of a lower social and intellectual background, whom he met intermittently. Although Mr. Black claimed to enjoy most of his homosexual activities, he had been impotent in attempting to assume the male role in intercourse, something he very much wanted to do.

The patient usually felt guilty after a sexual encounter, ostensibly for being homosexual instead of heterosexual, and frequently experienced the criticism as coming from the therapist. However, Mr. Black tended to attribute his guilt to violating social norms and not at all to the underlying aggression that accompanied his sexual experience.

This tendency was most clearly seen in the transference when he alternately fantasized the therapist's seducing him or vice versa. In either case, there was a prominent destructive component in which one of them sadistically inflicted pain and punishment on the other. At one point the patient reported a fantasy of being the devil and having sex with God and followed this with a series of associations of being like Samson in his super-masculine strength and destructiveness. This barely concealed transference fantasy in which he sexually attacked and subjugated the therapist was precipitated by his feeling that the therapist was trying to get rid of him by pushing him along faster in his treatment than he could go.

The expectation by the predictors that the patient's diffuse intensity, his patchwork self, would be an area of therapeutic exploration was quite accurate. The central issue that emerged midway in treatment concerned his elaborate and frequent masochistic masturbation activities that were his current major sexual outlet. The usual fantasy was that of being the sexual slave to a handsome, powerful male who forced him to endure a variety of painful sexual indignities. The main gratification was in feeling uniquely chosen by this superman to be his sexual partner, thus feeling needed and desired. After becoming indispensable, the patient turned the tables and then became even more powerful than his master. This fantasy represented a central transference paradigm that only gradually emerged and one that the patient had struggled to keep out of the therapy relationship. Essentially he was saying that he was willing to tolerate the indignities imposed on him in the treatment as long as he could maintain the feeling that he was uniquely important and necessary to the therapist. Only by means of resolving or modifying this defensive sadomasochistic fantasy (i.e., gaining love through submission and control) was this man able to attain a more positive self-image and greater freedom from depression, not to speak of the gratifying intimate relationship for which he was striving.

Mr. Black's sexual masochism, enacted in his masturbation activity but not in his sexual relationships, was part of a generalized masochistic orientation. He compared psychotherapy to the experience of crawling on a floor over broken glass with no respite in sight. He saw the therapist as wanting him to stay in a craven, obsequious, and suffering position so that he could enjoy the pleasure of feeling superior to the patient. Mr. Black recalled the childhood experience of having been beaten by his father and the perverse pleasure he had derived from the beating. Sadomasochistic love is better than none at all.

Painful suicidal ideation, which recurred with some frequency for the first few years of treatment, at first was primarily an expression of hopelessness associated with the major losses he had experienced in recent years. Subsequently, his suicidal thoughts represented a masochistic turning of his anger against himself, a way of protecting his ego ideal of the saintly, Christ-like person, while reinforcing his sense of moral superiority over those who are ruthlessly cruel. Coloring all this was his despair over failing to find a way of expressing his sexual wishes in a healthy open way that would be acceptable to him and to others.

The counterpart to his saintly self was never far from consciousness. Mr. Black also saw himself as diabolically destructive with inordinate wishes to retaliate and destroy those who made his life miserable. As a child he came to believe that he was the cause of his mother's fatigue and irritability, and he frequently had the idea that the therapist would like to be rid of him, indeed precipitously dump him. The patient often compared therapy to a chess game, with each opponent trying to see how clever he might be in triumphing over the other. His envy of the therapist's ability to understand him, which he equated with the therapist's power, led him at times to want to defeat the therapist and the whole therapeutic process, even if the patient was the main loser.

During much of the treatment, the work consisted mainly of dealing with the patient's view of relationships as basically fraught with the danger of being disappointed, demeaned, and ridiculed. He had extreme difficulty in thinking about an interaction with others in which mutually rewarding results could ensue. Mr. Black viewed every important negotiation in treatment as a win-lose situation, with the inevitability of him or the therapist emerging as the conqueror gloating over his helpless victim. These issues emerged with particular clarity in the course of certain necessary rearrangements in the treatment structure: reductions in frequency of appointments, charges for missed appointments, and coordination of vacation schedules. In each of these exchanges, Mr. Black had an opportunity to explore his resistance to discussing the problem; his fantasies of the expected outcome; and subsequent to a decision, the fantasied effect on the relationship. Over time he developed a greater conviction that equitable arrangements were possible and that authority figures would not necessarily attempt to abuse their power.

At each step in his giving up the hospital and partial hospitalization, Mr. Black felt that the therapist was robbing him of a treasured protection, while at the same time realizing that he had long since outgrown his need for such help. These occurrences provided the opportunity to look at his view of the therapist as "the enforcer," a reason for his fear of trusting a fully committed relationship to the therapist alone. It was not until the fourth year that the patient gave up an infrequent contact with an aftercare counselor who symbolized for him a safety net lest the therapist tire of him or suddenly show his "true colors" and terminate therapy. This characteristic of clinging symbiotically and parasitically to adjunctive supports while enjoying a generous insurance policy often created the most difficult countertransference problems for the therapist. The patient wanted to hold on much longer than he needed to, and his provocation to make the therapist into a depriving figure was often difficult to resist.

As these problems were clarified gradually and diminished in intensity, the patient's improvement took a quantum leap at the end of the fourth year when he was appointed to a teaching position commensurate with his professional training and competence, a job that he had believed to be essentially closed to him because of his sexual orientation. Until that time, Mr. Black had been preparing for a new career in an artistic endeavor and doing some private tutoring. His productivity, self-acceptance, and self-esteem were substantially increased, and he became considerably more accepting of his homosexuality. The reductions in treatment frequency were done at the patient's initiative, although not without some intense but short-lived anxiety. His marked improvement was an example of moderate intrapsychic changes associated with a diminution of his sadomasochistic conflicts, leading to adaptive life changes that in turn enriched the patient's sense of personal fulfillment. More succinctly, to rephrase an old saw, adaptive behavior was its own reward.

Termination became a serious topic of discussion in the last

6 months of treatment. Mr. Black felt that his life was proceeding satisfactorily, particularly in the success he was experiencing in his new position. In the sphere of relationships, he had not found a stable sexual partner but was still hopeful of doing so in the future. He still was not able to perform successfully as the penetrator in anal intercourse but felt that he had made progress in this direction. Also notable was a reduction in the frequency of his retreat into autoerotic activities, and even more significant was the virtual disappearance of the lurid sadomasochistic fantasies that formerly accompanied his masturbation, replaced by fantasies of mutually satisfying sexual activity. He continued to seek such a relationship in contrast with his past pessimism and reluctance to take the initiative in pursuing that goal.

The patient first opted for a tapering off rather than working toward a full termination. He had the idea of shifting to every other week and eventually to once a month, and so on. The therapist suggested that thinking in terms of a definite termination might be better, insofar as that would encourage the patient to deal more definitely with some difficult separation issues. Having a definite termination date was also a way of giving him permission to begin thinking about separation as a nonhostile action. For the first few weeks after having selected a date, Mr. Black had some return of symptoms, including his sense of hopelessness and suicidal ideation, which were interpreted as a manifestation of his anger about being shoved out. A detailed discussion ensued about his tendency to cut off abruptly relationships that have ended, with the feeling that the other person was not really interested in him anyway. A brief flurry of seeking transient sex was the patient's way of conveying that he needed further help. As the termination progressed, however, these issues subsided, and the patient was able to express genuine appreciation for the help he had received and sadness about giving up the relationship.

The technical approach in this treatment was a consistent focus on the transference, starting fairly early in the treatment. The predictors accurately delineated the areas of uncovering, including his "savage superego" that was manifested by his perfectionism, masochism, and suicidal ideation. Also, the patient's patchwork self, his as-if characteristics, and his oscillation between the extremes of all-good and all-bad were major areas of work. The patient's relatively recent loss of his father, the dissolution of his marriage, and the infrequent contact with his children were dealt with, particularly in the earlier phases of the treatment. As anticipated by the prediction group, structural change occurred in that Mr. Black became a more forthright and assertive person, consistent with the resolution of his underlying sadomasochistic conflicts.

In addition to the uncovering interpretative work, confrontations were sometimes brought to bear in relation to the patient's vagueness in the service of distance taking. Confrontations also addressed his efforts to avoid fully committing himself to the therapeutic relationship via his clinging to certain ancillary staff members longer than was necessary. But the prediction team's expectation that the patient's narcissistic vulnerability would require "structuring, reality confrontation, and advice . . . to help the patient to control his tendencies toward impulsive, ill-advised, and self-destructive behavior" did not occur as anticipated. Mr. Black was able to keep his impulsive acting out and his self-destructive behavior down to a minimum. In part, this may have been due to the long period of concomitant support that the patient received during the first half of his psychotherapy, first in the hospital and later during his partial hospitalization. In relation to his narcissistic vulnerability, the therapist offered self psychology interpretations (i.e., genetic explanations for the patient's infantile and narcissistic strivings) in an effort to become more explicitly empathic.

Assessment of Outcome

About 1 year following termination, two clinician-judges viewed the treatment outcome as very successful, particularly in terms of integration of grandiose/devalued self, reliance on more adaptive defenses, and a better modulated superego (see Appendix B, pp. 200–201, for more details on outcome assessment). These changes are captured by the improvement in the consensus rating on the Global Assessment Scale from 42 (serious symptoms or serious impairment in functioning) at the beginning of treatment to 71 (mild symptoms or some difficulty in functioning) at follow-up. Changes of similar magnitude occurred on the Bellak Scales of Ego Functions (Bellak and Goldsmith 1973) (see Appendix D, Table D–4) and on the Level of Functioning Scale (see Appendix D, Table D–1) devised by Waldinger and Gunderson (1987).

The judges noted the following kinds of structural, intrapsychic changes:

- The patient's infantile needs for nurturance are less intense and less infused with rage, therefore more adaptively expressed and satisfied interpersonally.
- He is far more tolerant of his needs and feelings, and his superego is much less severe, resulting in less masochistic or depressive submission to superego pressure. He has internalized the therapist's benign attitude toward himself and is consequently less dependent on others for external approval.
- Grandiose and devalued self-images are far better integrated, resulting in a more benign identity with less vacillation between masochistic submission and sadistic domination.
- The patient shows considerable insight into his symptoms and character pathology, particularly masochistic qualities and self-sabotage, as well as the narcissistic character defenses that previously precluded adaptive dependency on others. Rather than using his insight to impress others or keep them at bay, he uses insight to modulate his mood and behavior. The one area in which insight did not develop was in his attitudes and relationships with women.
- At termination, the patient was more capable of viewing the therapy as a partnership rather than a battle. Anger at the therapist was still largely expressed indirectly in behaviors geared to provoke the therapist to become the enforcer/depriver mother.

Also, the positive change in the patient's DIB scores from the beginning to the time of follow-up was instructive. Whereas the initial consensus score was 5, the outcome consensus score was 2. A significant event emerged in the interview that had occurred during the year-long follow-up period—he achieved his goal of establishing a stable sexual relationship with another man. Five years afterward, Mr. Black and his friend were living together in what appeared to be a mutually satisfying life.

Effect of Interventions on Collaboration

The consensus judgment of our six-clinician team was that 75% of the shifts in the alliance could be clearly related to interventions by the therapist (see Appendix A, chapter note 1).

The vast majority of shifts (89%) were in an upward (improved alliance) direction. This finding reflects a trend within most of the individual sessions, involving a gradual increase in the patient's collaboration that accompanied the therapist's clarifying, confronting, and interpreting transference elements. The majority of the positive shifts (63%) were related to interventions that focused on the transference relationship.

A vignette from the transcript may be useful in illustrating how transference interpretation increased collaboration. In session 728, near the end of treatment, Mr. Black is talking about a man he met. He is attracted to this younger man, but he is concerned that he will not be able to penetrate him if anal intercourse becomes a possibility between them. He then talks about a meeting he attended in which codependency and addictive behaviors were being discussed. He notes that some of the individuals involved were making excuses for why they did not change their behavior. He then reflects that he felt he did not have everything done as he approached termination. At this point, the therapist intervenes.

Tx: Well, in a way it seems to me that you were communicating last week, and now this week, parts of your life that have not changed or not changed enough, that you still would like to see get changed. And that sounds like it's also some kind of communication to me about possibly the incompleteness of the work . . . or maybe there are other things that are being communicated.

In this interpretation, the therapist focuses the patient's concerns on a transference issue, namely, that Mr. Black feels the therapist has left some of the work unfinished. Mr. Black responds to this interpretation as follows.

Pt: Yeah, I suspect that part of me, it's like with the termination coming, uh, you know, there's a part of me that wants to hang on to that and preserve that. So I don't know how much this stuff

[upward shift]

is . . . well, I know that this, the issues are real. Uh, I don't know in addition to that how much of that is, is a kind of a . . . either a, a plea or a manipulative kind of try to say, now, wait a minute, I'm trying to find some way for you to say, well, maybe we'd better continue . . . continue this for a while. Uh, which is, I'm, you know, it's pretty clear that part of me wants that. Uh . . . another part of me, I don't know, feels that, you know, the work we've done . . . uh, has . . . provided the process, uh . . . my, my internalizing and adopting of a process for dealing with my issues, and it's like no matter when we stop, I'm still going to have unresolved issues, uh . . . so I need to, to recognize that and . . . and in the time that remains working with you work on those issues as much as is possible and then, you know, continue to work on them on my own.

As indicated by the notation of upward shift in the margin, Mr. Black appears to increase his collaboration with the therapist. Instead of talking about external relationships, Mr. Black reflects on the interpretation and speaks more directly about his fears of termination and his disappointment in the incompleteness of the work. He also acknowledges his longing that the therapist would ask him to continue. The therapist's interpretation is clearly a contributory factor in the patient's upward shift in collaboration.

Transference interventions just as clearly played a key role in producing negative changes in the collaboration. All four of the downward shifts that could be linked to the therapist's interventions were in response to transference-focused comments. This finding confirms the well-known clinical wisdom that a transference intervention must be well timed, empathic, and worded in such a way that the patient can understand and assimilate the essence of it. Indeed, when transference interventions caused the therapeutic alliance to deteriorate, the researchers often noted that the comment was too direct, too long, too confrontive, or unempathic.

A good example of how a transference interpretation decreased collaboration can be found in session 526. The patient tells the therapist that he called the therapist's office on Memorial Day to make sure that it was a holiday and he would not be meeting with his therapist that day. He goes on to say that he feels he is not cared about. He longs for times gone by when people had loving relationships with each other. He cynically says that he does not believe that anymore. The therapist responds to these comments with an interpretation.

Tx: But it goes along with this whole idea of perfection, that either people are perfect and never do anything wrong to each other and they are always considerate and kind, or they are just the reverse and are just self-seeking and selfish and would just as soon get rid of other people. And it's like your feelings about yourself and feelings about me fluctuate from the idealized to the devalued, the good and evil. And it takes . . . it doesn't take very much, like it takes this kind of holiday, and talk about the holiday, to make you feel like I'm no good and I let you down and I don't even care about you and then a corresponding feeling of wanting to die (i.e., kill yourself) to show how I've let you down. A revenge type of thing.

The researchers generally agreed that the therapist's interpretation was too direct, too confrontational, not sufficiently empathic, and too long for the patient to assimilate fully. Even if the content were more or less accurate, Mr. Black may well have felt scolded by the tone of it. We now examine Mr. Black's response to the intervention.

Pt: Yeah, and I think one of the things that just distresses me about it is that it doesn't take very much to set off that kind of reaction, and I think, like I was saying earlier, one of the things I was trying to say about this, you know, sensitivity that I've always heard I've got so much of, it distresses me that it . . . things that normal people can take within stride, and I can't. It's like *I* was a lot more upset yesterday about D.'s mother being sick than he was. And it's like, you know, what the hell is going on here that I get so scared and distressed by that kind of thing and . . . and because at least the feeling that I have is that I know that a wish to die is a way to want to strike back at you, but *I* feel that it would be a mistake to see it only as that, because I think there is [down- a very strong feeling that I just wish it was all over, and if there ward shift] were some way that I could do it, without it having to reflect badly on you and without having to hurt my sons and make things difficult for them . . . that's what I would opt for because it . . . it just . . . it would just mean all this hurt will finally go away . . . and I think I'm . . . I'm . . . as I was saying earlier about not wanting to have a quick or a long-term cure or get better is because I guess deep down I feel so convinced that even by getting better it's like I'm never going to achieve, I guess, this degree of perfection that I feel I ought to achieve, either to be worthwhile or I want to achieve in order to be really able to accomplish the revenge that I want to accomplish.

The therapist's interpretation appears to have a negative impact on the patient's collaboration and elicits suicidal wishes. Mr. Black denies the importance of the therapist's intervention and is clearly at odds with the therapist when he says, "*I* feel that it would be a mistake to see it only as that." In other words, instead of making use of the therapist's interpretation, he is partially rejecting it but also struggling with it.

If one carefully studies the 32 upward shifts in collaboration that could be linked to the therapist's interventions (see Appendix D, Table D–3), a pattern emerges over the course of the treatment. In the first half of the treatment process, transference-focused interventions, including interpretation, confrontation, encouragement to elaborate, and clarification, seemed to be instrumental in producing the increase in collaboration. In the last half of the treatment process, however, *nontransference* interventions seemed to have been most contributory to upward shifts. In the last two or three sessions, the patient's collaboration was once again improved by transference-focused comments. The possible reasons for this change are discussed in the next section.

The overall competency rating of the therapist's interventions varied only slightly throughout the treatment. The lack of variability is not too surprising. First, the therapist was a senior clinician with a good deal of experience in treating borderline patients. Second, the lack of wide fluctuations in the patient's ability to collaborate also contributed to the therapist's consistent competency. Greater variations in competence are more likely when dramatic shifts in the patient catch the therapist off guard and erode the therapist's analytic "work ego."

Discussion

In this section we focus primarily on those factors within the patient that disposed him to make good use of an exploratory, uncovering therapeutic approach. Before presenting these findings, however, several issues require further attention.

Diagnosis

Since Mr. Black reacted to treatment in a manner more reminiscent of a neurotic than a classically borderline patient, we should consider the possibility of an incorrect diagnosis, both in his intensive week-long diagnostic evaluation and in his initial diagnostic studies as an inpatient. He did not show any clear intrusions of primary process thinking, nor was there good evidence of splitting in his interactions with others. As noted earlier, the consensus rating of 5 on the DSM-III-R criteria was reached by the research group.

The borderline diagnosis was based on a marked identity diffusion and pathological superego functioning. Mr. Black was described as experiencing himself as a patchwork combination of masculine and feminine, strong and weak, good and evil. He seemed to bounce actively from one side of each polarity to the other with little modulation. His primitive, indeed savage, superego was peopled by internal tormentors, such as a relatively personified God and Satan locked in battle, which disposed the patient to marked depressive reactions with suicidal ideation. The consensus judgment of the research team was that the patient met the following DSM-III-R criteria: unstable and intense relationships, potentially self-damaging impulsive behaviors, affective instability, recurrent suicidal threats, and marked persistent identity disturbance.

The research team, as well as the patient's treatment team, agreed on a borderline diagnosis and further concluded that he was a *high-level* borderline patient. Our conceptualization follows that of Meissner (1984), who viewed the borderline diagnosis as spanning a spectrum from high to low level, the former close to the neurotic border and the latter close to the psychotic boundary. Both Meissner (1984) and Kernberg (1975) believed that many of these high-level borderline patients are amenable to psychoanalysis or to a modified analytic approach. The efficacy of a highly expressive approach with this patient also supports the findings of the Kris Study Group (Abend et al. 1983) regarding the suitability of some borderline patients for analytic treatment. The significance of the fairly long period of hospitalization during his psychotherapy in making the expressive work possible is examined shortly.

As mentioned earlier, the consensus rating at follow-up on the DIB, a score of 2, had moved well out of the borderline spectrum. We believe that the structural change associated with a successful course of psychotherapy effectively boosted the patient out of the borderline range and that his functioning was now well within a neurotic range.

Developmental Factors

None of the relevant developmental factors constituted extraordinary traumas in the patient's past. Except for his mother's ongoing negative attitude toward males as sexual beasts and his father's need to be absent frequently from the home, the patient's developmental history included no early traumatic experiences nor sexual abuse nor neurological dysfunction.

Ego Factors

Motivation for change. The patient was highly motivated to find an accepting and affirming parental figure who could accept him despite his primitive urges, his dependency, his sadomasochistic wishes, and his homosexuality. At the same time, his harsh primitive superego produced considerable psychic pain, depression, and suicidal ideation, making it necessary for him to be treated initially with hospitalization and medication, but the negative affects provided him with a strong impetus to find relief through a better understanding of himself.

Capacity to work in an analytic space. Ogden's (1986) notion of "analytic space" is useful in understanding why Mr. Black did well with an essentially expressive process. Derived from Winnicott's

(1971) concept of "potential space," this construct connotes a particular way of thinking about experience that is conducive to psychoanalytic or psychotherapeutic work. Ogden defined this concept as "the
space between patient and analyst in which analytic experience (including transference illusion) is generated and in which personal
meanings can be created and played with" (p. 238). Mr. Black, for example, was usually able to experience transference perceptions as simultaneously real and not real. In other words, he was able to
perceive the therapist "as if" he were someone else without forgetting
that he was also a psychotherapist paid to help him. Even when the
therapist was experienced quite negatively, Mr. Black maintained an
observing ego that allowed him to differentiate external from internal reality. He was able to draw parallels between how he was experiencing the therapist at a particular moment and how he experienced
similar figures in his past in the same manner. Mr. Black was *not*
prone to psychotic transference distortions in which he would fall
into a paranoid-schizoid mode of relatedness, characterized by a collapse of analytic space and the experiencing of transference distortions as though they were "real" rather than "as if."

Impulse control and affect tolerance.   Despite the patient's marked
identity diffusion, severe superego pathology, a thought disturbance
that was evident both in clinical examination and on projective tests,
and a proneness to use primitive defensive operations, Mr. Black nevertheless had some notable areas of ego strength that contributed to
his ability to use expressive psychotherapy. He was able to delay
impulse discharge and modulate his affective states so that he could
reflect on the therapist's comments rather than take flight into
action, as is typical of lower-level borderline patients. As noted
before, his capacity for reality testing helped him to avoid slippage
into psychotic transferences and to maintain the analytic space in the
process.

Proneness to externalization.   Although many patients with borderline personality disorder tend to externalize their difficulties or
blame others for them, Mr. Black had the capacity to perceive his difficulties as arising from within. Even though he periodically would
perceive others as sadistically mistreating him, his predominant ten-

dency was to heap blame on himself. He believed that the other person would not be engaging in such mistreatment of him if he were a more worthwhile person. The parental admonishments that he recalled from childhood of having been told that he was responsible for the punishments meted out to him apparently became very much a part of his own thinking. Indeed, his past experience constituted the basis for the triad of masochistic-depressive-suicidal symptoms. Although some clinicians suggest caution about prematurely interpreting transference distortions because the patient is not ready to take back and own his projections (Epstein 1979), our patient showed a flexibility in his use of these projective tendencies. Part of the therapeutic work was to uncover his repressed and suppressed hostility, but his preferred style of directing aggression against himself rather than against others made him receptive to interpretations that spoke to his aggressive reactions and his tendency to internalize them. For example, his tendency to expect unfair, abusive treatment from the therapist could be interpreted both in terms of his early experience with his parents as well as a projection of his own aggressive impulses. He was amenable to seeing himself as the container of anger and the wish to inflict hurt partly because of his proneness to internalize.

Psychological-mindedness.   The patient had the capacity to think abstractly and psychologically about the issues brought to his attention. He became quite adept at translating metaphors into meaningful aspects of the transference relationship.

Relationship Factors

Narcissistic vulnerability.   Therapists of borderline patients often describe the feeling of having a very small margin of error in which to offer interpretations (Solomon et al. 1987). Lower-level borderline patients may react with explosive affect or flight when they feel an interpretation is unreasonable. Mr. Black, on the other hand, did not create the sense of having to "walk on egg shells" in delivering interpretations. Because of his need to maintain a positive relationship with an idealized male figure, and perhaps because of his internalizing tendencies as well, he would maintain a receptivity and tolerance of interpretive work. This receptivity, in turn, allowed the therapist to have a greater freedom to use interpretations.

Mirroring and idealizing transferences.   Idealization was a prominent feature of the work with this patient. Although perhaps partly related to a developmental arrest as described by Kohut (1977), the defensive aspects of Mr. Black's idealization were considerably more prominent. He attempted to flatter his "super therapist" as a way of lulling the therapist into inactivity. The patient used idealization as a defense against unacceptable aggression and competitiveness as well as a means of fostering his masochistic relationship to a therapist who would grow to depend on him for gratification. Mirroring needs were certainly present but were not overtly expressed; rather, he was alert to the therapist's interest in and commitment to him and was readily convinced that he could not trust the therapist's reliability.

Distancing and counterdependency.   The patient used his obsessional defenses to remain detached in the initial phases of treatment. His fear of closeness and involvement because of his mistrust and narcissistic vulnerability made him keep a safe distance. Gradually, however, he was able to overcome those fears, and his powerful wishes for closeness became evident.

Clinging and symbiotic needs.   Mr. Black experienced a considerable drive to find parental acceptance, approval, and affection. In his work he had always sought out positions in which he was in the shadow of an idealized senior male figure. He had some vague awareness that he was trying to improve on the disappointing relationship he had had with his own father. Mr. Black was able to experience some degree of warmth from his father, very much in contrast to his experience of his mother, but he was unable to develop a stable conviction that his father really loved him. The transference work provided the patient with the gratification of feeling pulled into a closer relationship with the therapist, even when the therapeutic work uncovered hostile content.

Sadistic and erotized transference.   The patient showed intense sadomasochistic wishes that constituted a major part of the therapeutic work. Evidence that these structures began to subside became apparent primarily in the shift in his masturbation fantasies, which became gradually more focused on mutual gratification with a sexual partner.

Capacity for concern. Mr. Black showed considerable ability to function within the depressive position, where he demonstrated a significant capacity for concern about others. From the standpoint of the structural model, his superego, although harsh, was sufficiently integrated to permit him to be concerned about his ability to harm others, and he would defend against it through the masochistic turning of aggression inward. Although certainly pathological, this high degree of depressive anxiety also made him more amenable to exploratory work than if he had functioned in a predominantly paranoid-schizoid mode, as is the case with many other borderline patients.

Flexibility Hypothesis

A significant patient characteristic involved Mr. Black's tendency to fluctuate between a desire for closeness and a need for distance. He was not committed to a polarized condition at either end of the continuum. As Horwitz (1985) noted, transference work may be compromised if the patient is incapable of moving flexibly within the closeness-distance spectrum. Mr. Black was not a clinging, dependent patient who wished to remain symbiotic and undifferentiated, nor was he one who experienced transference interpretations as redefining the boundary between the therapist and the patient, making it less permeable. Neither was he a patient who rigidly adhered to a remote, schizoid way of relating and who experienced transference interventions as intrusive and a violation of his self-imposed isolation.

Therapeutic Approaches

Assessing collaboration. Clinically, Mr. Black showed evidence of an increasing capacity to collaborate with the therapist over the course of the treatment. Slowly, and almost imperceptibly, he permitted the therapist to become an important and reliable person in his life, and as his sadomasochistic conflicts were interpreted and worked through, he became less fearful of the therapist's power to damage or destroy him (see Appendix A, chapter note 2).

Pattern of interventions. Most writers on the psychotherapy of borderline patients subscribe to the idea that active uncovering interpretive work, especially with regard to the transference, should be delayed until the patient has had an opportunity to develop a somewhat stable, trusting relationship (i.e., a therapeutic alliance). The findings with this patient, however, are somewhat at variance with this recommendation. We discovered that the therapist began using transference interpretations early in treatment, and, in fact, in the latter half of treatment transference interpretations decreased, although the work was just as expressive (see Appendix A, chapter note 3).

We believe that the decreased use of transference interpretations in the latter half of the treatment can be explained on the basis of two factors. First, Mr. Black's anxieties about closeness and his fear of being sadistically abused by the therapist led him to engage in obsessional soliloquies, smoke-blowing obfuscation, and other distancing devices. To make meaningful affective contact with him in the early stages of treatment, the therapist found that actively interpreting the patient's transference resistances was necessary.

A second factor is that the patient began to internalize the therapist's mode of working within the transference and began doing such work largely on his own. As early as session 194, in the second year of treatment, the researchers noted the patient's spontaneous references to the transference that were connected with two upward shifts. By the middle of the treatment, the therapist found that drawing the patient's attention back to the transference was unnecessary because the patient was able to do that for himself. One possible explanation for the return to the transference focus in the last two or three sessions is that the patient's flight from dealing with his grief around termination resulted in the therapist's having to draw Mr. Black's attention back to the loss of the relationship with the therapist. A frequent observation has been the return of initial symptoms at the end of a long-term psychotherapy. Similarly, the patient's initial defensive pattern of flight from the transference may have returned as the treatment was ending.

Other technical considerations.   Particularly in the early sessions, before the patient had become accustomed to the idea of working with the transference, the therapist's persistence in pursuing this approach seemed to be useful. This does not mean, of course, that one should single-mindedly plunge ahead with all patients who are made uncomfortable by transference interpretations. But the therapist believed that Mr. Black had the potential to tolerate such work. Also helpful was the therapist's making explicit that content to which the patient could only hesitantly allude. The therapist's ability to perceive and verbalize the patient's indirect hints at difficult content, especially sexual and aggressive references, often granted the patient permission to pursue these matters further. The therapist's style of exploration, which often consisted of statements like "let's try to understand this better," enhanced the therapeutic alliance.

The research team was frequently struck by the "benign cycle" in which therapist and patient mutually built on each other's contributions. The more the patient demonstrated a willingness to explore his inner world, the more the therapist felt free to communicate his observations and understanding. These were occasions of an escalation of openness and collaboration that we often associate with "the good hour."

Another significant factor that may have contributed to the patient's amenability to an expressive approach was the patient's hospitalization and partial hospitalization. The patient was hospitalized on an extended-treatment unit of a psychoanalytically oriented hospital for the first year and a half of the psychotherapy. Particularly in the first year of the treatment, if hospital protection and support had not been available, the therapist's uncovering work may not have been tenable, partially because of the persisting suicidal threat the patient presented. It was also clear to the therapist that Mr. Black required other significant people in his treatment at the outset before he could commit himself to the relationship with the therapist. The patient may only have been willing to take the risks of exposing himself in the therapy because of his awareness of having a support system of other treaters, first on the hospital unit and later in the partial hospital program.

Countertransference. The chief countertransference reaction was the therapist's difficulty in tolerating the patient's sense of entitlement. Because of his more than adequate insurance benefits, the patient pressured his treaters to extend his hospital stay for a longer period than was absolutely necessary. In general, Mr. Black was loath to give up any of his treatment benefits, and this constituted an irritation to the therapist, particularly when the other treaters acceded to the patient's wishes.

Summary

The patient was a high-level borderline man who began psychotherapy while still a hospital patient. He had developed a marked depression with suicidal ideation after the breakup of his marriage, primarily associated with his homosexuality. Also, a troubled relationship with his principal was threatening to lead to the termination of his position as a high school teacher. The first 2½ years of psychotherapy were conducted while he was a hospital or partial hospital patient, and for the remaining 4½ years he was essentially an outpatient. The psychotherapy was conducted, for the most part, at three times a week and was predominantly an expressive treatment. The patient's marked improvement in his depressive symptoms and in his acceptance of his homosexuality was based largely on an attenuation of his harsh superego and his sadomasochistic character, which had disposed him to seeking tense, subjugated relationships with authorities, with the fantasy of becoming indispensable to them.

The following characteristics contributed to Mr. Black's amenability to an expressive, uncovering approach:

■ The high-level nature of his borderline personality disorder was helpful in the sense that he showed relatively good impulse control and frustration tolerance, although he suffered from identity diffusion and a patchwork self of contradictory self-images concealed by an as-if veneer.

■ His depressive tendencies spoke to a relatively strong internalizing tendency, in contrast to a more externalizing-paranoid orientation, and this characteristic lent itself to looking inward and uncovering unacceptable aspects of his self.

■ His need to experience empathic attunement with a parental figure, while disposing him to being a compliant as-if personality, also contributed to greater efforts by the patient to collaborate with the therapist in the uncovering process.

■ In terms of the flexibility hypothesis, this patient was not committed to a polarized position with regard either to a desire for closeness or to a need for distance. Instead, he flexibly shifted from one orientation to the other, facilitating a long-term expressive treatment.

References

Abend SM, Porder MS, Willick MS: Borderline Patients: Psychoanalytic Perspectives. New York, International Universities Press, 1983

American Psychiatric Association: Diagnostic and Statistical Manual of Mental Disorders, 3rd Edition, Revised. Washington, DC, American Psychiatric Association, 1987

Bellak L, Goldsmith L: The Broad Scope of Ego Function Assessment. New York, Wiley, 1973

Epstein L: Countertransference with borderline patients, in Countertransference: The Therapist's Contributions to the Therapeutic Situations. Edited by Epstein L, Feinder AH. New York, Jason Aronson, 1979, pp 375–405

Gabbard GO, Horwitz L, Frieswyk S, et al.: The effect of therapist interventions on the therapeutic alliance with borderline patients. J Am Psychoanal Assoc 36:697–727, 1988

Gunderson JG, Kolb JE, Austin V: The Diagnostic Interview for Borderline Patients. Am J Psychiatry 138:896–903, 1981

Horwitz L: Divergent views on the treatment of borderline patients. Bull Menninger Clin 49:525–545, 1985

Kernberg OF: Borderline Conditions and Pathological Narcissism. New York, Jason Aronson, 1975

Kohut H: The Restoration of the Self. New York, International Universities Press, 1977

Meissner WW: The Borderline Spectrum: Differential Diagnosis and Developmental Issues. New York, Jason Aronson, 1984

Modell AH: The "holding environment" and the therapeutic action of psychoanalysis. J Am Psychoanal Assoc 24:285–307, 1976

Ogden TH: The Matrix of the Mind: Object Relations and the Psychoanalytic Dialogue. Northvale, NJ, Jason Aronson, 1986

Solomon MF, Lang JA, Grotstein JS: Clinical impressions of the borderline patient, in The Borderline Patient: Emerging Concepts in Diagnosis, Psychodynamics, and Treatment, Vol 1. Edited by Grotstein JS, Solomon MF, Lang JA. Hillsdale, NJ, Analytic Press, 1987, pp 3–12

Waldinger RJ, Gunderson JG: Effective Psychotherapy With Borderline Patients: Case Studies. New York, Macmillan, 1987

Winnicott DW: Dreaming, fantasying, and living: a case history describing a primary dissociation, in Playing and Reality. New York, Basic Books, 1971, pp 26–37

Ms. Green

Ms. Green, a divorced woman in her early 30s, began psychotherapy 3 months into hospitalization on an extended inpatient treatment unit. Transferred from a short-term unit where she
had been hospitalized in the midst of a crisis, the patient had a long
history of alcohol and drug abuse, impaired impulse control, and destructive behavior. She had been treated by many psychiatrists since
late adolescence, with multiple brief psychiatric hospitalizations in
conjunction with outpatient psychotherapy and pharmacotherapy.
The crisis hospitalization that preceded the referral for extended inpatient treatment was precipitated by assaultive behavior during an
episode of intoxication.

Ms. Green was a member of a family that had suffered many tragic
losses. Her early development was shaped by hyperactivity. In addition to high activity levels, she showed periods of head banging. Most
problematic was her refusal to go to sleep. Her parents went to great
lengths to get her to go to sleep, including staying up with her until
the early morning hours. When this was ineffective, her pediatrician
prescribed barbiturates. Even when she was staggering from the medication, she would not go to sleep. In desperation, her parents finally
wedged the door shut and left her alone in her room. She was enraged
and screamed herself to sleep. Although her extreme hyperactivity
abated, she remained a highly active child.

Notwithstanding this early history of developmental difficulty,

Ms. Green did well socially and academically in her early school years. In the beginning of adolescence, however, she began to show more disturbed behavior. She became rebellious, and her parents felt that she was uncontrollable and emotionally out of reach. She began a pattern of severe polydrug abuse, including alcohol and a wide range of prescription and street drugs. A significant trauma was the loss of a very close friend who died in an accident. She was able to graduate from high school, and she attempted college, earning good grades at times, but she was unable to sustain academic work with any consistency. She also worked at a number of jobs, but she was not able to support herself consistently and hence remained financially dependent on her parents. Intertwined with continuous drug and alcohol abuse (including many blackouts) were emotional lability, destructive relationships, antisocial activity, and reckless behavior (e.g., driving while intoxicated, automobile accidents, a boating accident that resulted in serious injury).

The social worker who met with the patient's family during her hospitalization described Ms. Green as having alarmed her parents for several years. They were unsuccessful in finding adequate professional guidance, and they characteristically gave in to her demands for support despite her continuing destructive behavior—notwithstanding heated confrontations. Ms. Green typically sought treatment from psychiatrists who would prescribe drugs she craved, and her parents continued to finance such treatment, despite their serious misgivings about it. The social worker characterized the parents as intelligent and kind people who had not received adequate professional help, and she noted that a good treatment alliance with both parents was readily established. Indeed, the parents steadfastly supported the extended inpatient treatment, despite the patient's repeated protests and demands for discharge.

Psychological testing conducted soon after Ms. Green's admission to the hospital revealed a somewhat contradictory picture of assets and deficits. Ms. Green was seen to fit the "classical description of the borderline patient," with a need for immediate gratification, sensitivity to abandonment, a self-destructive way of rebelling, and a proclivity to engage in power struggles and protracted battles in relationships. She showed a complex character structure, with indications of histrionic and antisocial features. Moreover, she showed some ca-

pacity for delay and modulation of impulses and well-preserved reality
testing. The psychologist who tested Ms. Green also noted the significance of her history of drug abuse in addition to the borderline disorder, underscoring the fact that Ms. Green had had some chemical
in her system every day for many years. Her verbal IQ was 21 points
higher than her performance IQ, and this led to a referral for neuropsychological testing, which revealed erratic cognitive functioning as
well as deficits in left-right discrimination, spatial orientation, visuospatial and semantic memory, and fine-motor coordination, along
with difficulty shifting cognitive sets. The patient's cognitive deficits
were seen to reflect an amalgam of long-standing neurological impairment compounded by substance abuse and psychological conflicts.
Verbal and abstract reasoning skills, as well as a good vocabulary, had
all been preserved. Her good verbal skills tended to obscure her cognitive impairment, which was revealed only on formal testing.

With her affective lability, cognitive impairment, chronic and severe substance abuse, and multifaceted character structure, Ms. Green
presented a complex diagnostic picture. She had been given a diagnosis of bipolar disorder in previous treatment, but she had not had
a sustained period of drug-free functioning, and the putative mood
disorder was therefore confounded with drug abuse. During a long
period of relatively drug-free functioning in the hospital, there was
no further indication of a diagnosable mood disorder, although
Ms. Green continued to be emotionally labile, partly in the context
of premenstrual syndrome. Her primary diagnoses at the time of discharge from the hospital were attention deficit disorder without hyperactivity and borderline personality disorder. Despite her history
of severely maladaptive behavior, she had significant assets. The social
worker was optimistic about treatment, for example, commenting that
she was a beautiful young woman with many social skills, an attractive
and appealing manner, and high intelligence.

Predictions

Two senior clinicians who had no knowledge about the course of
treatment assessed Ms. Green, using the initial data to predict the
optimal treatment strategy. The following is a summary of their consensus judgments.

The judges emphasized Ms. Green's extreme sensitivity to loss and abandonment, evident in "the ease with which her perceptions of abandonment, loss, and separation trigger panic, the experience of being lost in life, and attempts to seek restorative drug experiences. Her need to surround herself with admiring others reflects a failure to achieve object constancy." More specifically, she had developed an expectation that relationships will eventuate in violent and painful endings. "A core issue likely to pervade much of the treatment involves the theme in Ms. Green's life, and that of her family, of loss or abandonment as a result of violent action. This is reflected in the family history and in the accident that killed her close friend."

The judges saw Ms. Green as likely to oscillate between the extremes of closeness and distance. She seeks the stimulation, danger, and excitement that relationships can provide, but she takes distance when not immediately gratified or uses drug states to provide distancing numbness. She plays this out in such ways as overdependence on parental supports, alternating with periods of aloof detachment. These extreme oscillations in relationships are determined largely by environmental factors, turning in particular on how containing and benignly structuring the situation is. The proclivity to vacillate was coupled with a history of superficial relationships. "On the one hand, she seems to act out, in a driven fashion, clinging, symbiotic attachments involving high-intensity, danger/thrill-imbued experiences. Yet, there is not a sense of enduring emotional attachment or reciprocity in these relationships, which do convey a significant as-if quality."

The judges predicted that Ms. Green would benefit most from a highly expressive treatment, albeit with a moderate degree of supportiveness. Thus they saw the need for interventions to be focused predominantly on the patient-therapist relationship, with less emphasis on nonrelationship issues. They gave the following rationale for an expressive approach: "We sense a greater potential for self-control, psychological-mindedness, and introspection in her than she shows at first glance. Her social adaptation shows promise for her developing a capacity for utilizing a therapeutic alliance for more expressive work." While recommending this treatment approach, they were aware of Ms. Green's potential aversion to support. "She seems to take some strong satisfaction in not receiving supportive measures. This appears in part to represent masochistic gratification but also seems to have some qualities of nonmasochistic pride in being able to tolerate a more stringent form of treatment." They listed several treatment issues as needing expressive work: loss and abandonment, masochism, rage over unfulfilled dependency needs, narcissistic emptiness and perfectionism, and a harsh superego evident in expectations of punishment and self-punitiveness.

Although the judges recommended a predominantly expressive approach focusing on the patient-therapist relationship, they also articulated several technical problems with the implementation of such an approach based on Ms. Green's limitations. These included "her defective insight masked by pseudo-sophistication and compliance; her impulsivity and ego-syntonic acting out; her dependency masquerading as motivation; complications brought on by her neurological impairment; and the ever-present potential to abruptly flee treatment because she 'is cured' (a flight into health) or, perhaps, a flight into jail."

Ms. Green's cognitive impairments were anticipated to be an obstacle to effective interpretation. The judges stated that the patient's cognitive vulnerabilities—especially when anxious—could cause her to become overwhelmed when asked to engage in the kind of synthesis involved in interpretation. They also indicated that the treatment, at times, would need to shift in a supportive direction because of her exquisite sensitivity to actual or perceived loss, and consequent extreme emotional reactions during times of turmoil. She was seen as likely to withdraw emotionally from the therapist as experiences of closeness intensified and, at such times, to require supportive interventions to quell the anxieties as they arose in the treatment relationship. She was also seen to need empathic attunement by the therapist to assuage her fears that relationships would be damaging, praise to bolster her self-esteem, and advice to deter destructive action.

The complexity of the diagnostic picture is paralleled by the apparent contradictions in the treatment recommendations. Despite numerous indications for supportive measures and several cautions about an expressive approach, the judges came down on the side of an expressive emphasis in the treatment. In light of the severity and chronicity of Ms. Green's characterological disturbance, the judges concluded that nothing less than an ambitious treatment approach would have a substantial impact. For example, they recommended that confrontation be used "with caution at first and then 'ruthlessly' later on." In effect, the judges concluded that the treatment could potentially move in an increasingly expressive direction and that an expressive approach would stand the best chance of generating improvement. Moreover, the judges based their prediction in part on a transcript of one of the initial psychotherapy sessions, at which point Ms. Green's collaboration was relatively good.

Course of Therapy

Ms. Green began psychotherapy after 3 months of hospitalization. She was seen for a total of 207 hours over the course of 2⅓ years. She began at a frequency of twice-weekly sessions, increasing at her request to three times a week 2 months later. The patient remained in the hospital for a year after psychotherapy began, but soon after being discharged from the hospital to a partial hospital program, she requested a decrease in the number of hours (back to twice per week). Several months thereafter, concomitant with her dropping out of the day hospital program, she unilaterally decreased the frequency of therapy to 1 hour per week, a frequency that continued until her termination.

Ms. Green began hospital treatment and psychotherapy showing relatively little insight into her illness; she was prone to see her difficulties exclusively as revolving around her being a "drug addict." At the same time, however, she frequently viewed the only help she could get as being in the form of pills to relieve her distress. She regularly declared her intention to leave treatment, often in a self-destructive fashion (e.g., planning to leave in such a way that her insurance coverage for subsequent hospitalization would be jeopardized). Ms. Green remained very attached to her previous psychiatrist, whom she characterized as readily yielding to her demands for tranquilizers and with whom she described a rather informal, friendly relationship. Often, she berated her hospital psychiatrist for withholding medication and for confronting her with her psychological problems. Keenly ashamed of her previous self-destructive behavior, she felt humiliated when, as part of her hospital treatment, the destructive behavior was brought up in the presence of other patients in the treatment group.

Ms. Green began by idealizing the psychotherapist, and she frequently split her hospital psychiatrist and psychotherapist in her mind, seeing the former as depriving and persecuting and the latter as more benevolent and understanding. The therapy began with a honeymoon phase, in which Ms. Green expressed an interest in psychotherapy, opened up a great deal about her past behavior about which she felt extremely guilty, and experienced some relief in being able to talk openly about herself. At this early juncture, Ms. Green's functioning in the psychotherapy process appeared somewhat consistent with the capacity for expressive work that the judges making the predictions had envisioned. Yet, she also began with considerable trepidation. She was concerned about confidentiality and initially feared that the tape recordings done for research purposes would be made available to her hospital treatment team. She also feared that the psychotherapist would reveal secretive behavior to her hospital doctor that might result in her freedom being curtailed. The therapist forthrightly told the patient that the content of the psychotherapy would remain confidential unless he became concerned that she was at risk for seriously harming herself.

Soon after beginning psychotherapy, however, Ms. Green's experience of the psychotherapist began to fluctuate, concomitant with her fluctuating moods. She felt comforted, at times, and expressed satisfaction in being understood. At other times, she perceived the therapist as frustrating, cold, and unhelpful. She longed for her former psychiatrist and would urge the psychotherapist to intervene with her hospital psychiatrist to obtain more medication for her. The patient often felt profoundly empty and at times appeared walled off from the therapist. Feeling empty, her only recourse was to impulsive action, and at such times it was difficult to obtain any sense of what was going on inside her or to conduct much psychological work. Indeed, her penchant for externalization ultimately carried the day. As it turned out, the therapist was unable to sustain an expressive approach.

Ms. Green's ambivalence about the psychotherapy came to a head several months into the process in relation to the therapist's annual vacation. She requested a substitute therapist for the duration of several weeks. This request was granted because she appeared to be able to make use of the neutrality afforded by the opportunity to talk more openly with a therapist who did not have administrative responsibility for her hospital structure. On her regular therapist's return, Ms. Green declared that she wished to transfer to the substitute therapist. She found him more comforting, humorous, and supportive, and she reported that he offered her much-needed advice. She also thought that the substitute therapist would be more supportive of her leaving the hospital soon. The substitute therapist also reminded Ms. Green more of her previous psychiatrist. Subsequent exploration suggested that Ms. Green's relationship with the substitute therapist was more like her easy-going preadolescent relationship with her father, whereas her feeling about her regular therapist was more like that about her father in her adolescence (i.e., experiencing the therapist as more withdrawn and critical). Her wish to transfer appeared to repeat a long-standing pattern where, when rejected by one man (i.e., her regular psychotherapist going on vacation), she immediately found another (the substitute therapist) to fill the void. Although declaring a wish to transfer therapists, Ms. Green flatly stated that she essentially wanted *no* treatment, describing her use of the hospital as a "resort." The therapist took a neutral stand regarding the transfer, advocating exploration and understanding prior to a decision. Ms. Green ultimately decided not to transfer, stating that she wished to preserve the work that had already been done with her regular psychotherapist.

The patient's conflicts with closeness in relation to men were also evident in the fact that, while on passes from the hospital, she established a romantic relationship with a man in the community, a relationship that was also marked by oscillations in closeness and distance. For a period, she appeared to be alternating in her attachments to her boyfriend, her hospital psychiatrist, her former psychiatrist, her psychotherapist, and the substitute psychotherapist.

Ms. Green also oscillated in her relationship with her parents. Characteristically, she resented their not responding empathically to her. She came to recognize, however, that her rebellious, angry retreat had obstructed any possibility of their helping her. Moreover, the patient felt extremely guilty for the anguish she had put them through. She was reluctant to explore her feelings about her parents in the past and in the present, for the most part blocking that area of work. Her parents' consistent support of hospitalization felt like a rejection to her, and the patient often felt as if she had been dumped in the hospital "like trash." Yet, examination of any negative feelings toward them often made her feel profoundly disloyal. At one point after an altercation with her boyfriend, she eloped from the hospital, traveled to the distant eastern city in which her parents lived, and spent the weekend with them. Ms. Green appeared to be testing her parents to see if they would still accept her, despite her anger toward them, and to see if they would insist on her return to the hospital—they passed both tests.

Throughout the middle period of treatment, Ms. Green consistently played out a split. She angrily declared her wish to leave the hospital, against medical advice if necessary, rebelling against the controls and restrictions imposed by her hospital psychiatrist. She attempted to maneuver the psychotherapist into a position at variance with that of her hospital team, urging him to consent to further psychotherapy outside the hospital, despite the hospital team's objections. The therapist took the stand that he would not agree to see Ms. Green outside the hospital without a workable posthospital treatment program. While remaining on the extended-treatment unit, she was referred to a daytime program for substance abuse, in part to begin to prepare her for discharge, when she would be at highest risk for relapsing. This was a positive experience in the sense that she developed the firm conviction that substance abuse was dangerous for her (the patient had surreptitiously abused drugs in the hospital at times prior to that). Yet, another split developed as the psychiatrist in the substance abuse program viewed her as needing little additional hospitalization, in contrast to her hospital psychiatrist on the extended-treatment unit. Another major struggle ensued, as she demanded to be discharged from the hospital sooner rather than later, despite her regular psychiatrist's stance that she needed additional hospitalization, the substance abuse program psychiatrist's opinion notwithstanding. The psychotherapist took the middle ground that, if Ms. Green were insistent on leaving the hospital, she should first agree to have a remaining period of hospitalization entailing much more autonomy to test herself further before discharge. Ms. Green agreed to work toward discharge with this understanding.

A key relationship paradigm was becoming increasingly evident: Ms. Green disavowed her dependency and insisted on autonomy. Yet, she did so in a way that raised alarm and invited others to hang on tight and exert considerable control. She then felt persecuted and mistreated, fought, and was prone to break off the relationship, only to find another in which the pattern was repeated. In maintaining a counterdependent stance, she was able to externalize her difficulty onto those who were controlling her. When the hospital treatment team and psychotherapist became unified in an autonomy-granting stance (albeit with some continued hospitalization and planned discharge to a structured day hospital program), the target of her struggle shifted. Ms. Green began to feel overprotected and excessively controlled by her parents, who began to show apprehensions about her functioning outside the hospital. Throughout this period, Ms. Green's continuing penchant for action and externalization tended to preclude expressive work in the psychotherapy.

About a month before she was to be discharged from the hospital, Ms. Green requested to listen to the research audiotapes for the purpose of reviewing and reflecting on her progress. Several sessions were devoted to listening to several audiotapes spanning the many months of psychotherapy. Her collaboration during this period was excellent; she was insightful about the material in hindsight, and she also brought in material that she had censored earlier. Ms. Green found it particularly meaningful to hear a tape of a session early in the psychotherapy process in which she had come in after taking diazepam. In retrospect, she found her denial to be astounding. The confrontation with her denial about the seriousness of her substance abuse provided by the tapes proved especially helpful. Notably, after the agenda of listening to the tapes was completed, Ms. Green felt a void and had little sense of inner problems to work on in therapy. Listening to the tapes had been gratifying, had provided structure, and had provided an external focus, all of which she subsequently missed. Without the task of reviewing the tapes, she turned her attention back to another external focus: leaving the hospital and cutting down treatment.

Even before Ms. Green was discharged, she requested a decrease in frequency of psychotherapy sessions, repeating her counterdependent stance. She consented to wait until after discharge before making the change but continued to insist on decreasing sessions after she left the hospital. The therapist reluctantly agreed because he saw no other option. Soon after she left the hospital, Ms. Green repeated the pattern of wanting to break away in relation to her partial hospitalization. Her participation in the day hospital program was inconsistent, and she also missed a number of psychotherapy sessions. Yet, for a time after she left the hospital, she was able to use the psychotherapy productively. Although she continued to rebel against controls, the extent of externally imposed control was markedly decreased, and the basis for her externalization was substantially diminished.

Accordingly, Ms. Green began to explore her long-standing conflicts with men and her long-standing pattern of destructive relationships. She saw that not all of her erratic and destructive behavior was related to drug abuse. She recognized her conflicts with authority. Experiencing moments of overwhelming anxiety about her capacity to find and hold a job, she was able to face her distress rather than self-medicating. She could also acknowledge significant problems with having low self-esteem, wanting to be perfect, and being hypersensitive to criticism. She even began to appreciate her tendency to alarm others when she was in the process of separating, and she began to recognize a sense of dependency on the psychotherapist. She again requested a substitute therapist during her regular psychotherapist's vacation, although this time she made good use of the substitute therapist without any disruption in her relationship with the regular psychotherapist.

As Ms. Green continued to move in the direction of further autonomy, however, the treatment again became progressively problematic. She had obtained a job and had begun to develop considerable success in the work arena. Yet, she concomitantly sought to decrease her involvement in treatment (i.e., day hospital), again externalizing her difficulties onto the partial hospital treatment team and battling in relation to her structure. Disavowing her difficulty in letting go, Ms. Green sabotaged the discharge process in such a way that the treaters continued to hang on to her, prolonging the termination process.

Ultimately, Ms. Green was discharged from the partial hospital program. Her progressive withdrawal from treatment was also evident in the psychotherapy. She frequently missed appointments and often rescheduled her appointments because of the demands of her job. Presenting the therapist with her unilateral decision, Ms. Green declared that she was decreasing therapy to once a week. She viewed this decision as absolutely mandated by the external reality of her job, not subject to negotiation or exploration. In effect, the therapist had the options of reducing the sessions or terminating the treatment. The therapist acceded to the reduced frequency. She continued to miss a number of appointments even at the reduced frequency. The patient used the therapy as a source of support and stability, but she showed little interest in any exploratory work. She was functioning relatively well, maintaining a demanding job, and establishing a network of friends. She periodically visited her family and was pleased about her relationships with them. By this time, however, she had resumed fairly regular use of marijuana.

As Ms. Green decreased her involvement with psychotherapy and treatment more generally, she became even more intensely involved with her boyfriend (i.e., moving in with him). Her relationship with him had been fraught with ambivalence from the outset, but the problems escalated. She characteristically focused on her boyfriend's dependency on her, his inclination to control her, as well as his unreliability, while minimizing her dependence on him. She began to think about ending her relationship with him as well as terminating her psychotherapy. In the psychotherapy, she was acknowledging her dependency somewhat more, while simultaneously becoming increasingly disengaged.

Consistent with her history, Ms. Green ended both relationships in a stormy fashion. The possibility of a smooth termination was aborted by a major crisis. Ms. Green felt rejected by her boyfriend, and after a major altercation with him, she became severely intoxicated such that emergency hospitalization was needed. Once admitted, Ms. Green immediately declared her wish to leave the hospital. She was discharged with the understanding that she would continue psychotherapy, resume contact with her former hospital psychiatrist (who treated her during the emergency hospitalization), and find a more suitable posthospital structure. She did not attend the next scheduled psychotherapy appointment and subsequently telephoned the therapist to notify him that she had gone to live with a friend on the East Coast. Ms. Green did not resume psychotherapy, but she continued to telephone the therapist periodically, sometimes during periods of crisis, and at times during transitions and significant events in her life.

Assessment of Outcome

Two clinician-judges examined the initial, termination, and follow-up data to rate the changes in Ms. Green about 4½ years following termination. The follow-up material included repeat psychological testing and a videotaped interview (Diagnostic Interview for Borderline Patients [DIB] [Gunderson et al. 1981]). It is important to note that the psychotherapy was not completed. During what was planned as an extended termination phase, Ms. Green prematurely ended psychotherapy in a sudden and unanticipated flight from the area. Nevertheless, the judges viewed the treatment outcome as relatively successful, with limited but significant improvement noted in most areas of psychological functioning. In contrast to her functioning at the time of termination, by follow-up Ms. Green had markedly reduced substance abuse and self-destructive behavior. Nevertheless, she remained in need of relationships in which blame could be externalized and conflicts acted out. The changes over the course of her treatment are captured by the improvement in the consensus rating on the Global Assessment Scale from an initial score of 36 (i.e., major impairments in several areas) to 55 (i.e., generally functioning with some difficulty) at the time of follow-up. Similar changes were indicated on the Bellak Scales of Ego Functions (Bellak and Goldsmith 1973) and on the Level of Functioning Scale (see Appendix D, Table D–5 and Table D–8) devised by Waldinger and Gunderson (1987).

The judges noted the following intrapsychic and behavioral changes at follow-up, 4 years after termination:

- Ms. Green's vulnerability to peremptory demands for gratification were considerably reduced; however, her reduced dependency on others was largely a function of increased suppression and denial.
- She was less occupied with a view of herself as grossly defective and was, therefore, less depressed and less prone to self-destructive behavior.
- Her identity, formally based more on antisocial allegiance to drug culture, was now more established in her role as mother and worker.

■ Although Ms. Green was even less reflective and psychologically minded than at the outset of treatment, she seemed better able to avoid grossly destructive life circumstances. At the beginning of treatment, she was experiencing far more pain and subjective distress; at the end, her defenses and denial were strengthened.

■ Ms. Green had come to view the therapist as an ally and auxiliary ego who could be contacted on an "as-needed" basis.

The positive change in Ms. Green's DIB scores from the initial interview to follow-up was informative. Whereas the initial score averaged across raters was 6.5, the score at follow-up averaged 4.5. This 2-point drop reflects a shift from near the cutoff point, indicating a borderline diagnosis, to well below that point. A significant series of events emerging in the interview was Ms. Green's rather abrupt and premature termination of her treatment and her subsequently becoming reestablished in another community. She developed an enduring—albeit conflictual—relationship with a man, gave birth to a child, and assumed responsibility for the care of her child, while also maintaining productive outside employment.

Effect of Interventions on Collaboration

The majority of shifts that could be linked to the therapist's interventions (68%) were in the upward direction (improved alliance). However, only a minority (29%) of these upward shifts were related to interventions that focused on transference. These findings reflect this patient's frequent lack of positive response to transference interventions and the relatively greater weight of supportive interventions. Occasionally, a transference interpretation was fruitful but primarily when preceded by multiple supportive interventions.

Perhaps more impressive than the trend for Ms. Green to fail to show positive alliance shifts in response to transference interventions was another more persistent form of resistance. When Ms. Green was experiencing strong affect, intent on a course of action or presenting a particular argument or point of view, any effort by the therapist to encourage exploration or greater reflectiveness was typically met with avoidance or denial. Ms. Green's alloplastic orientation and her preference for externalization and action over exploration persisted as the primary line of resistance over the duration of the therapy.

To illustrate various factors bearing on Ms. Green's use of the therapist's interventions, we have chosen three vignettes.

An example of the difficulty encountered in encouraging Ms. Green to assume a self-critical reflective stance appears in session 161. Ms. Green came to the session in an agitated state, saying that she had come from a fight with her boyfriend and complaining that she had hurt her thumb when she slammed her car door. The therapist supported Ms. Green's scheduling an appointment with an internist to examine her thumb, and then Ms. Green continued to voice her complaints against her boyfriend.

Pt: He is! He is, he's just, he's just nuts. You know, he really is. He's he's never going to get any better if he hasn't by now. [sniffs] The only thing I can do is remove myself from it so he won't keep tearing me apart. Do you think I'm wrong? I mean, am I over-reacting?

Tx: Oh, no. It seems normal to me to be very upset when you're attacked.

Pt: [sniffs]

Tx: I don't see that you're crazy, it just seems that you're very upset.

Pt: [sighs] And I am worried about work. And, you know, he doesn't have a job, of course he should help me with things. When I didn't work, I prob . . . first of all, you know, I ran the dry cleaning, you know, I did everything, I ran all his errands. I paid his bills, I called credit, you know, I mean [gulps] when one isn't working, one handles those things, it's just understood, you know, it's like I told him, when, when, when the real estate business was, was so bad, my uncle, you know, my uncle's wife worked, and my uncle took care of everything. That's how it is. [sniffs, sighs]

Tx: I wonder if there's still a bit of something in you that's inclined to hurt yourself, you know? I mean, not consciously, but, you know, if you get mad or if you're attacked, it seems like you did injure yourself . . .

Pt: I know.

Tx: or get careless with yourself. I gather it makes you mad at . . .

[down-
ward
shift]

Pt: I just don't know what I, I mean, I don't even want to analyze it. . . .

Tx: [sighs, clears throat]

Pt: You know, it's like I've got. I can't be around him. I don't know what I'm going to do! [tearful]

Tx: Well, there's some, there's something, though, that goes on inside you that I think is important to be aware of, and that it is you get mad at yourself.

Pt: [sniffs]

Tx: Maybe tend to blame yourself for what's happened.

Pt: [sniffs] If I have to get a cast on this, which I think I will, will I have to do that here? Do they do stuff like that here or will I have to go to the hospital?

The downward shift in the margin indicates that Ms. Green decreased collaboration with the therapist. When the therapist attempted to help her acknowledge the self-destructiveness in her behavior, she stated, "I don't even want to analyze it" and thereafter ignored the therapist's interventions. Nor had there been much indication in the prior work that Ms. Green was in a frame of mind to examine the meaning of these events.

The next excerpt is from session 32 and illustrates the difficulty in helping Ms. Green work with transference-focused material, particularly negative transference. The level of collaboration throughout this session had been low and sinks lower as Ms. Green places responsibility for her transference-based feelings onto the influence of drugs.

Tx: Um-hum. Maybe you're feeling, uh, kind of disengaged now?

Pt: Yeah, that's a very good word for it. It's just, it's strange 'cause when you say things, you know, I can tell that they're true but when you ask me to give an example, I can't really think of one.

Tx: Um-hum. See, I think, uh, one . . . one way you have of becoming engaged with me, for example, is by being angry.

Pt: Wh-When did I . . . become angry . . . with you? I don't under-stand what you mean by that.

Tx: You can't recall being angry with me?

[wn-ward hift]

Pt: That on . . . that, but that was . . . because I had taken drugs . . . that one time.

Tx: Uh-huh, yeah, that wa . . . well, that's a prime instance . . .

Pt: Yeah.

Tx: as I remember you saying at the time that you were feeling in a way good about what was going on.

Pt: Um-hum. Well, when I took drugs here, it just, you know, it just, I don't, I don't know how to describe it, it just, uh, made me more aware of how I was feeling.

Tx: Um-hum. But it's not only then. You were feeling . . . angry a week ago, so angry that you felt like you were on the verge of leaving. And you were quite angry at me mainly because you felt I was misunderstanding you. By emphasizing my vacation as a part of that. You're feeling more disengaged today than usual?

Pt: Yeah, I really am.

Tx: Any idea why that would be?

Pt: I just am so tired of being around so many people. It's just the intensity of it. You know, I just . . .

The downward shift in the margin represents the predictors' con-sensus of a probable negative shift in the alliance. They were able to predict that this patient's response to a focus on negative transference, particularly her anger with the therapist, would be avoidance and ex-ternalization.

The final example is from session 129, which shows Ms. Green's tendency to respond with an improved alliance to therapist interven-tions that were supportive and empathic. In allowing Ms. Green, in part, to externalize responsibility for that which was negative, the interventions also allowed Ms. Green to acknowledge some of her own problems. This excerpt begins with Ms. Green's discussion of her stormy relationship with her father and parallel difficulties with her boyfriend.

Tx: He did hurt you and you hurt R. in a kind of similar way . . .

Pt: Um-hum.

Tx: . . . to how your father had hurt you.

Pt: You know, I mean, it's like my mother when she tries to make people feel guilty, you know, I—I do something, something similar . . .

Tx: Um-hum.

Pt: . . . to it too.

Tx: Um-hum.

Pt: And it's funny, today I was thinking driving over here, it's a good thing I'm not in Providence because I really felt for the first time I would love, there's this one bar in Providence, it was an outdoor cafe . . . was not a bar, it was a restaurant, very nice restaurant, that I'd love to just go in and have some drinks. But, uh, you know, the feeling passes. That's why I—I don't act on it.

Tx: Um-hum. Because of the tension you were feeling?

Pt: Yeah.

Tx: Um-hum.

Pt: Yeah. And th-the thing that's so fun—it would not work anymore, you know, that's what I tell my parents. You know, I—I couldn't do it again . . . because I'm not, I'm not mentally like I used to be.

Tx: Um-hum.

Pt: And it just, it wouldn't work anymore. That to me isn't even an option.

Tx: Um-hum. Well, it certainly is to your credit that you're managing to face all this tension now . . . that you used to dispel.

Pt: Um-hum.

Tx: But it isn't easy.

[ward
shift]
Pt: Well, therapy, it's just, God *I hate to think of you leaving town,* I really do. Um, 'cause it's really been a help for me and I'm glad I will have a substitute therapist because a lot of it is just keeping in the habit of doing that.

Tx: Um-hum.

Pt: You know, because as busy as I've been I, you know, I've always made sure I've gotten here.

Tx: Um-hum.

Pt: You know, and it's not out of no sense of obligation like a lot of times I'd say boy if I wasn't in the hospital and I wasn't afraid of not getting charted, you know, I . . .

Tx: Um-hum.

Pt: It's, you know, because I—I find, I find a lot of comfort in it. Well.

The cumulative effect of the therapist's helpfulness and, in particular, the therapist's praise of Ms. Green ("it certainly is to your credit") contributed to Ms. Green's feeling that the therapist was helpful and to her concern about his absence and finally to the upward shift in the alliance. It is also noteworthy that this shift consists of Ms. Green's elaborating on positive transference feelings, in contrast to her typical flight from discussing negative transference manifestations.

Discussion

The treatment process did not unfold as anticipated by the judges who made the predictions. Although the predictors delineated ample reasons to provide support, they recommended a predominantly expressive approach. The actual process was rated as only moderately expressive and slightly more supportive than expressive. In retrospect, several factors militated against a predominantly expressive approach. This discussion reviews the contraindications for an expressive approach that became clear in the course of treatment and describes the associated therapeutic strategy. The conclusions presented here reflect the consensus of the research team based on integration of the available clinical and research data.

Diagnosis

A comprehensive psychiatric evaluation conducted at the time of admission and an extensive psychological assessment were consistent in pointing to a borderline disorder. As stated earlier, the psychologist who conducted the testing concluded, "This is a young woman who, in many respects, appears to fit the classical description of the borderline patient." Ms. Green showed conspicuous splitting in her relationships, alternating between idealization and devaluation. She had pervasive problems with impulse control and engaged in severely self-destructive behavior, at times gravely endangering and seriously injuring herself. She had severe angry outbursts, had a markedly unstable sense of self and identity, and complained of chronic emptiness. Despite the severity of Ms. Green's symptoms, she could be considered "midlevel" in the borderline spectrum, because she did not show the psychotic regressions characteristic of the most severely disturbed borderline patients.

To confirm the clinical diagnosis, the six core research team members independently reviewed the initial clinical material and made a judgment as to whether Ms. Green met each of the eight DSM-III-R (American Psychiatric Association 1987) criteria for borderline personality disorder. There was a clear consensus that she met seven of the eight criteria (i.e., unstable and intense relationships, impulsiveness, affective instability, intense anger, identity disturbance, emptiness, and efforts to avoid abandonment—but not recurrent suicidal threats). Notwithstanding the consistency of the findings regarding the DSM-III-R diagnosis, the average of the six research team members' ratings on the DIB, based on the videotaped interview, was 6.5, falling just short of Gunderson's cutoff point (7).

Developmental Factors

Early trauma. Ms. Green was disinclined to explore her childhood experience of family relationships. In effect, her attitude was: "My parents treated me well—why should I have these problems?" Yet, a history of early traumatic experience was evident. She was so hyperactive in infancy that her parents, after going to extraordinary lengths to help her settle down, ultimately resorted to wedging her door shut and confining her to her crib such that she would be in a rage and eventually scream herself to sleep. Accordingly, unable to soothe herself or to feel soothed by others, she likely felt abandoned in a state of extremely high distress and arousal. Early in life, she had been prescribed sedative drugs as a means of regulating emotional arousal; later in life, she resorted to the same device.

Neurological dysfunction. Ms. Green's hyperactivity in early childhood likely was, in part, rooted in neurological dysfunction. Neuropsychological testing conducted as a part of her inpatient evaluation documented residual cognitive deficits consistent with those commonly found among patients with borderline disorders (O'Leary and Cowdry 1994). In all likelihood, these constitutional factors contributed to impairment in capacity for self-regulation. Ms. Green's severe substance abuse was an effort on her part to compensate for her inability to calm and soothe herself, but the substance abuse only further eroded her controls and the adequacy of her functioning.

Ego Factors

Motivation for change. Ms. Green's motivation for change was transitory, at best. She initially expressed some desire for insight and appreciation for insight, but she was far more prone to externalization, focusing her attention on the shortcomings and failings of others. She often chose action over reflection and persistently endeavored to flee treatment. She acknowledged that she had a history of extraordinarily turbulent and problematic relationships with men, but she attempted to resolve this by establishing a new idealized relationship with a man. When the idealization failed, Ms. Green resorted to externalization. Later in the course of her hospital treatment, she made good use of a program for substance abuse but tended to close off further exploration with her newfound identity as a "drug addict." She showed a period of relatively good motivation after she had dispensed with all treatment except psychotherapy; then she could not externalize problems as due to treatment, and she became more aware of her own shortcomings and low self-esteem. She was ambivalent about being in psychotherapy and eventually terminated abruptly.

Capacity to work in an analytic space.   In contrast to the first patient, Mr. Black, Ms. Green had great difficulty adopting a reflective as-if attitude regarding her experience. There was often a collapse of "analytic space" (Ogden 1986) because she was unable to take distance from her feelings and distorted perceptions of herself and others. Instead, Ms. Green often felt convinced of others' malevolence and her victimization. Often, and with conviction, she expressed hate for her hospital doctor, insisting that he was incompetent and destructive, rather than examining the internal basis for her feelings. Having at one point surreptitiously read her medical record, she declared that she was "borderline" and prone to "splitting." She was occasionally able to use this knowledge in an intellectual way to gain some detachment from her angry devaluation of her hospital doctor, but this awareness was short-lived.

Impulse control and affect tolerance.   Inherent in splitting is a diminution of ego resources, evident in Ms. Green's impaired capacity to regulate affect, delay impulse expression, anticipate the consequences of behavior, and perceive relationships accurately. As noted earlier, constitutional vulnerabilities, compounded by chronic and severe substance abuse, also contributed to ego weakness. Her impairment closely conforms to Grotstein et al.'s (1987) description of the most common clinical manifestation of borderline disorders: impaired self-regulation. This feature is observed in patients who fail in the capacity for self-soothing and soothing through object relations and, instead, turn to drugs, alcohol, or other self-destructive means of regulating discomfort and tension. Rather than verbalizing her feelings, reflecting on them, and finding comfort in such exploration, Ms. Green was prone to acting them out (e.g., in quickly establishing and maintaining a romantic relationship coincident with the onset of therapy, continuing episodic drug use, eloping from the hospital). At times, she was able to be more thoughtful—but often as a prologue to plunging directly into action. Her verbalizations were often akin to actions, inasmuch as she would threaten what she would do rather than reflecting on her need to act.

Proneness to externalization. Ms. Green consistently externalized her difficulties, blaming her treaters for her plight and dysphoric feelings. Her externalizations were rooted in splitting. Quite often, her hospital psychiatrist was the bad object, and the psychotherapist was the (relatively) good object. When the psychotherapist returned from his first extended vacation, he became the bad object and the substitute psychotherapist, the good object. Her parents shifted from good to bad, but Ms. Green predominantly tried to protect them from her negative feelings. She was extremely reluctant to examine the role of family dynamics in her own difficulty, a form of combined splitting and protectiveness that has been described as a major impediment to the constructive use of psychotherapy in certain borderline patients (Colson 1982).

Ms. Green revealed glimpses of severe guilt, which attested to the intensity of her depressive anxiety and her fear that her hate would destroy the few good objects she was able to preserve. Any comment by the therapist that Ms. Green construed as critical of herself or her valued relationships were met with avoidance, denial, and self-destructive action. Such reactions are reminiscent of Epstein's (1979) recommendation to contain and metabolize the borderline patient's projections and need for an external bad object, rather than interpreting the transference projections, thereby returning the bad-object projections to the patient.

Psychological-mindedness. The various factors just discussed that compromised her ego functioning contributed to Ms. Green's limited psychological-mindedness. Most notably, her penchant for splitting and externalization continually eroded her capacity for introspection and reflection, as did her tendency to cope by means of destructive action and flight. She showed periods of psychological-mindedness, but she was disinclined to sustain any self-examination and exploration.

Relationship Factors

Narcissistic vulnerability. Kernberg (1975) noted that one contraindication to an expressive approach with borderline patients is extreme narcissistic vulnerability. This was a factor of paramount importance in Ms. Green's psychotherapy. Her self-esteem was extremely low, and she felt profoundly ashamed of her past actions and her difficulties in functioning. She had very high aspirations and felt humiliated about being hospitalized, to her way of thinking, with a group of "low-functioning" patients. She was liable to feel humiliated when her problems were brought out into open in the hospital treatment groups. In the psychotherapy process, she experienced any exploration of the basis of her feelings and actions as a potential criticism. Any hint of criticism in an intervention tended to undermine her collaboration, whereas praise and recognition of her accomplishments had a more salutary effect.

Mirroring and idealizing transferences.   Although she made limited use of the therapist's efforts to promote insight and self-understanding, Ms. Green did make constructive use of the therapist's presence and efforts to understand and respond to her distress. At the outset of psychotherapy, she formed an idealizing transference in which she eagerly absorbed the therapist's interest and "insights." Then the therapy provided a comforting and soothing refuge from the split-off, persecutory hospital treatment environment. At times in the latter part of treatment, a mirroring transference was evident. Ms. Green took pride in presenting her relatively good functioning to the therapist, and she used his acceptance and affirmation to bolster a budding, more positive self-image. As the final vignette (session 129) illustrates, Ms. Green was able to use the therapist's empathic attunement to bolster not only her self-esteem but also her capacity for self-regulation; at the same time, the relationship served to maintain her sense of self-cohesion.

Distancing and counterdependency.   Ms. Green showed a pattern of counterdependence and avoidance throughout her treatment. Occasionally, she was able to acknowledge her dependency and to express gratitude toward caretakers. But she could not feel safe for long in a dependent position. She continually focused her attention on getting out of the hospital, often engaging in major battles in the process. Once out of the hospital, she immediately set her sights on getting out of her partial hospital program. Concomitantly, she insisted on reducing the frequency of her psychotherapy sessions.

Ms. Green's counterdependent stance, coupled with her vulnerability to self-destructive action, ensured that others, in fact, would not let her go. The harder and more violently she pulled away, the more she unwittingly invited treaters to hold on to and pursue her. For example, her vociferous demands for discharge from the hospital, in combination with continuing signs of impaired functioning, only confirmed her hospital staff's conviction that she needed to remain for extended inpatient treatment.

Clinging and symbiotic needs. Ms. Green tended to deny and externalize her need to cling to others. She deflected her dependency out of the psychotherapy by quickly establishing an intense relationship with a man in the local community. As previously stated, she maintained an overtly counterdependent stance. Yet, she would demand that others grant her more autonomy while simultaneously communicating that she was liable to do something dangerous or destructive. Accordingly, others would tend to hold on to her or refuse to let her go, and Ms. Green would perceive them as clinging to her. The same pattern was evident in her relationship with her boyfriend, inasmuch as she focused on his depending on her while dismissing her dependency on him.

Sadistic and erotized transference. Ms. Green did not express sadistic or erotized feelings or fantasies in her relationship with the psychotherapist. She kept the relationship relatively neutral and occasionally proclaimed that she did not have the expectable "transference." By virtue of splitting, Ms. Green preserved the psychotherapy relationship by keeping her aggression primarily focused on other relationships, those with her boyfriend and hospital psychiatrist. In those relationships, she tended to externalize her aggression and to feel mistreated and misunderstood. Her hospital doctor was seen as sadistic and persecutory. At other times, she became overtly hostile and aggressive in these relationships, particularly with her boyfriend. As illustrated by the vignette from session 32, Ms. Green was relatively unable to experience or reflect on her anger within the psychotherapy relationship. Yet, a partial enactment of a sadomasochistic relationship occurred in the psychotherapy insofar as Ms. Green, at times, tormented the therapist (i.e., raising his anxiety by embarking on destructive action) and felt tormented by him (i.e., by his pursuit and efforts to hang on).

Capacity for concern. Ms. Green's anger and attacks on others predominated in much of her treatment. Yet, she also demonstrated a capacity for concern that played a significant role in her benefiting from treatment. She felt guilty for the hardship and turmoil she had put her parents through, and she feared damaging them (e.g., their health) further. Ms. Green clearly recognized the destructiveness of her behavior, and she did not want them to suffer any further. She felt enormous gratitude for their support in the face of her anger and destructive behavior. Accordingly, her concern for them provided an important incentive to curb destructive impulses.

Flexibility Hypothesis

Ms. Green did not show a flexible shifting between closeness and distance. As mentioned earlier, she maintained a predominantly counterdependent stance throughout her treatment, although glimmers of a capacity to tolerate dependency were revealed for limited periods. Most often, she tended to maintain a relatively rigid distance, expecting to be attacked, exploited, and abandoned in a close relationship. As the predictors noted, a major theme is that of "loss or abandonment as a result of violent action." Ms. Green's termination of psychotherapy was strikingly consistent with this paradigm. A violent altercation ended her relationship with her boyfriend, and she abruptly terminated treatment soon thereafter. She took the active part in both ruptures, as she made an effort to avert the dreaded passive position of being abandoned.

Therapeutic Approaches

Assessing collaboration. Ms. Green's collaboration was relatively poor throughout the psychotherapy (see Appendix A, chapter note 5). At best, for brief periods, she made an effort to reflect and to use the process to understand herself. Most often, however, she was disinclined to be introspective, focused on current external problems, and tended to externalize. Over the course of the psychotherapy, Ms. Green's collaboration deteriorated slightly, as she gradually pulled away from the therapist. Also notable is the finding that, within sessions (i.e., from the first third of a session to the last third), she typically showed no improvement in collaboration. Thus, she was generally unable to use a psychotherapy session to become more reflective.

Pattern of interventions.   Ms. Green's therapy was characterized by an exceptionally high level of therapist activity (see Appendix D, Table D–6). The therapist's conversational style included a great deal of dialogue. There was a relatively high level of activity across types of intervention, although the proportion of interpretations was comparatively low, and exploration, affirmation, and confrontation predominated. Also, consistent with this supportive approach, the interventions were primarily focused on matters outside the patient-therapist relationship. More specifically, the therapist very actively attempted to clarify Ms. Green's thoughts and feelings as well as the events she was describing. The interventions were often directed toward clarifying her scattered, confusing, cryptic, and contradictory communications when she was emotionally aroused. The therapist actively intervened to maintain a focus, persistently pursuing a seemingly important issue in the face of Ms. Green's attempts to flee her feelings and conflicts. One member of the research group, after reading the transcript of one such session, commented that Ms. Green and the therapist were like "fighter planes, with the therapist in rapid pursuit." In addition, the therapist actively provided guidance and direction when Ms. Green felt lost or empty.

Also noteworthy (see Appendix D, Table D–6) is a dramatic shift in the nature of the therapist's interventions over the course of the therapy. Specifically, in the last third of therapy, the use of interpretation and relationship-focused interventions plummeted, because Ms. Green showed an inability to tolerate such an approach.

Often when therapists begin therapy with an expressive orientation, they may be averse to shifting to a more structured and supportive approach (Colson et al. 1985; Horwitz 1974). Ms. Green's therapist, however, managed to avoid that pitfall. Taking his lead from the patient, he became increasingly supportive, used a high level of activity, and proportionately reduced the focus on transference.

Other technical considerations.   The therapist adapted his style to Ms. Green's prominent needs for a soothing, holding relationship. In effect, he "held" her with a high level of engagement and verbal activity. This style dovetailed with her impaired capacity for self-soothing and self-regulation, coupled with her sense of vulnerability to abandonment. From what was learned of her history, she likely felt abandoned early in her childhood. She had been experienced as uncontainable, and she was ultimately confined alone in an extremely agitated state. Ms. Green's admission to the hospital was a dramatic repetition of this paradigm. She was in a state of high arousal, being withdrawn from drugs, and feeling abandoned by her parents and by her former psychiatrist (who had prescribed drugs). However, she was not left alone; her hospital psychiatrist stayed with her, and he tolerated her rage. In addition, the psychotherapist stuck with her throughout. Indeed, the therapist's extremely high level of activity in the therapy hours may have reflected his awareness of Ms. Green's predisposition to feel abandoned in the hour (Waldinger and Gunderson 1987).

Ms. Green was not abandoned; she was contained. There was no question in the patient's mind that the prolonged containment provided by her hospitalization was crucial. Indeed, years later, once she no longer was dependent on him, she regarded her hospital psychiatrist with affection and gratitude, appreciating the lifesaving effect of the containment he steadfastly provided.

Countertransference.   Ms. Green's high level of affect, and her readiness to act in self-destructive ways, repeatedly stirred the therapist's anxiety, such that the therapist also felt a need to *do* something (e.g., calm her, dissuade her from rash action), having difficulty himself maintaining a reflective posture. In effect, Ms. Green's agitation became contagious, and the therapist replayed the model of parental alarm, as if he were attempting to cajole a recalcitrant child. Projective identification was evident when Ms. Green calmly announced a self-destructive plan and the therapist anxiously attempted to dissuade her.

Other countertransference determinants of the therapist's high level of activity were evident. When she was not actively doing battle, Ms. Green often became depressed and explicitly complained of feeling empty. At such times, the therapist was drawn into activity, in effect, to fill the void. In addition, the therapist became embroiled in struggles for control, as implied by the fighter plane metaphor previously described. Ms. Green was often in a counterdependent mode, and the therapist endeavored to maintain some control, in effect, trying to pin her down.

The therapist was also partially drawn into the split with the hospital team, notwithstanding his desire to remain neutral. Ms. Green attempted to have the therapist become her good ally, protector, and advocate in relation to the bad hospital team, and she became angry and felt abandoned when he disappointed such expectations. Ms. Green's account of her functioning in the hospital was often more positive than the hospital team's account. The therapist was, at times, drawn into the middle (e.g., at one point advocating a compromise between Ms. Green's declaration that she would leave the hospital immediately and the team's insistence that she spend much more time in the hospital).

Also prominent in the treatment of this patient was a variant of "institutional countertransference" associated with the therapist's involvement in the research project. Notwithstanding that the project was explicitly designed with the assumption that some borderline patients are best treated supportively, in the therapist's perception, expressive work was most valued by the institution and by the research team in particular. In addition, the research was specifically directed toward focus on the nature of interventions that would enhance the alliance—obviously desirable. Ms. Green's continually problematic alliance did not go unnoticed by the therapist. Moreover, the research group's definition of the alliance was somewhat biased in the direction of expressive work. Consequently, reminded by the presence of the tape recorder, the therapist was aware that a given session might be scrutinized by the research team, and he feared that his inability to improve the faltering alliance would be criticized. Although the therapist's high level of activity was generally regarded as helpful, he sometimes appeared to be overly active, at worst, intrusively and angrily attempting to drag Ms. Green into an alliance in relation to expressive work. Thus, the therapist's sense of pressure in relation to the research agenda and his colleagues' scrutiny contributed counterproductively to an already high level of anxiety and emotional arousal in the process and the relationship.

Summary

Although the predictors advocated a primarily expressive approach to the psychotherapy with this patient, the actual process was only moderately expressive and slightly more supportive. Moreover, the therapy became increasingly structured and supportive over the course of the treatment, with the therapist taking his lead from Ms. Green's inability to tolerate or benefit from an interpretative focus. Such support was manifested both in the therapist's high level of verbal activity and his reduced focus on transference. Ms. Green's collaboration, never at a very high level, tended to deteriorate over the course of the therapy, but paradoxically she seemed to benefit significantly from the process.

Several factors mitigated against Ms. Green's constructive use of an expressively oriented psychotherapy. Her need for a supportive approach was rooted in a marked developmental disturbance. She demonstrated significant areas of ego weakness associated with constitutional vulnerabilities, evident in impaired self-regulation and her inability to soothe herself. Nor could she comfortably respond to efforts by others to soothe her; she feared interpersonal closeness, expecting to be attacked, exploited, and abandoned. Her narcissistic vulnerability, stemming from these developmental deviations and compounded by a history of profoundly destructive behavior, played a prominent part in the need for support. She often responded best to interventions such as praise, advice, recognition of accomplishments, and emphasis on the adaptive side of defenses. Expressive interventions were liable to heighten her narcissistic vulnerability, fueling her penchant to externalize. Consequently, she was unable to adopt a reflective as-if attitude to transference experiences, in effect, leading to a collapse of analytic space.

Ms. Green was ill equipped to make use of expressive psychotherapy, but she made good use of multiple supports. Most important, she had the experience of not being abandoned or exploited, but contained, in the hospital and in the psychotherapy. This was in dramatic contrast to her "uncontainable" affect and behavior that characterized much of her development from infancy to adulthood. She managed at least periodically to idealize the therapy as a place where she could obtain benevolent advice, praise, and soothing. Although she struggled mightily and continually to flee from treatment and to engage in self-destructive behavior, Ms. Green and the therapist managed to sustain the relationship. She was able to experience efforts to contain and metabolize her projections and to contain the anxiety associated with her self-destructiveness. She did not experience the retaliation she had come to expect in prior relationships. We would emphasize, however, our conviction that the psychotherapy relationship could not have been sustained without the containment provided by extended inpatient treatment and partial hospitalization, an option that has become increasingly rare.

References

American Psychiatric Association: Diagnostic and Statistical Manual of Mental Disorders, 3rd Edition, Revised. Washington, DC, American Psychiatric Association, 1987

Bellak L, Goldsmith L: The Broad Scope of Ego Function Assessment. New York, Wiley, 1973

Colson DB: Protectiveness in borderline patients: a neglected object relations paradigm. Bull Menninger Clin 46:305–320, 1982

Colson DB, Lewis L, Horwitz L: Negative outcome in psychotherapy and psychoanalysis, in Negative Outcome in Psychotherapy and What to Do About It. Edited by Mays DT, Franks CM. New York, Springer, 1985, pp 59–75

Epstein L: Countertransferences with borderline patients, in The Therapist's Contribution to the Therapeutic Situation. Edited by Epstein L, Feiner AH. New York, Jason Aronson, 1979, pp 375–405

Grotstein JS, Solomon MF, Lang JA (eds): The Borderline Patient: Emerging Concepts in Diagnosis, Psychodynamics, and Treatment, Vol 1. Hillsdale, NJ, Analytic Press, 1987

Gunderson JG, Kolb JE, Austin V: The Diagnostic Interview for Borderline Patients. Am J Psychiatry 138:896–903, 1981

Horwitz L: Clinical Prediction in Psychotherapy. New York, Jason Aronson, 1974

Kernberg OF: Borderline Conditions and Pathological Narcissism. New York, Jason Aronson, 1975

Ogden TH: The Matrix of the Mind: Object Relations and the Psychoanalytic Dialogue. Northvale, NJ, Jason Aronson, 1986

O'Leary KM, Cowdry RW: Neuropsychological testing results in borderline personality disorder, in Biological and Neurobehavioral Studies of Borderline Personality Disorder. Edited by Silk KR. Washington, DC, American Psychiatric Press, 1994, pp 127–157

Waldinger RJ, Gunderson JG: Effective Psychotherapy With Borderline Patients: Case Studies. Washington DC, American Psychiatric Press, 1987

Ms. White

Ms. White, a married woman in her early 30s and mother of several children, was acutely depressed at the time she sought an outpatient consultation. She found herself increasingly apathetic and unhappy about her life, yet she was apparently happily married, had a good job, and was pleased about her education and career. She was puzzled that she felt so miserable. She thought that she should be able to cope on her own but became frightened by her thoughts of suicide. She entertained the idea of slitting her wrists, yet she did not really believe that she would do so.

The patient was the oldest of several children born to her parents within the span of a few years. There had been chronic marital discord throughout most of her childhood. The basic needs of the children were met, but little warmth or affection was available. The patient was recruited to help care for her younger siblings at an early age and had become a parentified child. Family life was chaotic, without appropriate boundaries of many sorts. The patient had little privacy as a child in their small home, sharing one bedroom with two sisters. The fact that her parents were second-generation immigrants from impoverished and ethnically diverse backgrounds contributed still more to the discord and stress with which the patient and her family had to contend.

Ms. White's relationships with her siblings were distant and troubled at the time of the initial consultation. A younger brother had been depressed, self-destructive, and aggressive since adolescence, requiring numerous psychiatric consultations. A younger sister was even more troubled and had committed suicide 2 years before. Other siblings, although not as severely disturbed, experienced symptomatic and characterological problems serious enough to disrupt their adjustment.

The patient's depressive state intensified at the time of major holidays, when the absence of her sister had been glaringly obvious and painful for all. The suicide had exploded the myth that they were a close and warmly connected family and was followed by a period from which neither she nor other family members had recovered. The patient was overwhelmed with feelings of guilt as the parentified child, feeling that she had failed her siblings, and was overcome as well by her parents' grief.

The patient felt that she had been depressed most of her life but had become significantly worse following her sister's death. She had remained in bed crying, had no appetite or interest in life, and was barely able to function. She received a course of antidepressant medication (amoxapine) for 6 months, which gradually helped her to recoup and permitted her to return to work as a social worker in a nursing home specialty unit. The medication was discontinued a year before the patient began therapy. She found the medication very helpful, but she continued to be troubled by the fear that she would not be able to concentrate adequately. Despite the chronic family turmoil and lifelong depressive symptomatology, the patient had been able to complete her professional education and was working on an advanced degree.

For more than 5 years prior to the consultation, the patient had been bulimic, with a typical frequency of bingeing and purging once a week. Physically a healthy child, she had always been thin and was pressured since childhood by grandparents and parents to eat and gain weight. The bulimia began at the time of her move from her parental home and was recurrent, particularly under stress. For example, it often occurred at the end of a school semester when she felt the pressure to obtain good grades. She had been able to abstain from vomiting periodically but she retained the symptom, finding her bulimia difficult to resolve and even more difficult to reveal and discuss. She experienced a mixture of feelings about her vomiting: relief and pleasure at ridding herself of the food and what it represented but also loss of control and a loss of self-esteem.

Parental attitudes toward her seeking treatment were quite mixed. The mother could not believe that her healthiest child needed help; the father was supportive and empathic, acknowledging that she had never had a childhood, because she was needed to help them. She was stunned that he was that insightful and found it meaningful that he could share the observation with her. In fact, he proved instrumental in helping her to seek treatment. The patient's husband also was supportive. A stable, hard-working professional, he was tolerant, loving, and eager to find help for his wife.

Psychological testing was conducted soon after the inception of the psychotherapy. The findings were consistent with the diagnosis of borderline personality organization, confirming the diagnostic impression of the outpatient consultant. The psychologist noted that the patient's thinking was realistic and well organized when the tasks were clear and well structured. Nevertheless, serious lapses occurred under the pressure of her angry feelings, at which time she could become highly projective and illogical. There was evidence of identity diffusion in her contradictory and unreconciled self-images. Most prominent was a vision of herself as competent, serious, and nice—an image born out of compliance that excluded expressions of anger and fostered a sense of innocence. Ms. White was consciously fearful that to give up such an image would anger those important to her, who would in turn abandon her. Concomitantly, she tended to exaggerate her sense of being frightened and victimized to coerce others to remain attentive. Thus, she related to people masochistically, turning anger toward herself, suffering and hoping to be cared for. Although the patient craved nurturance, she was unable to experience genuine affection. Her proclivity for affective flooding and dyscontrol was highlighted in the context of her history of self-destructive action.

The testing psychologist noted a major developmental disturbance evidenced in the poor differentiation of self and object images in her projective test responses, with a thematic emphasis on concerns over separation. He felt the patient had the potential for a major depression with psychotic features and that she was in a state of decompensation related to her sister's death. In commenting on her characterological makeup, he underscored narcissistic and compulsive features manifest in her emphasis on appearance and her tendency to distance herself from others with a rigid investment in work.

Specifically, he emphasized her problems in regulating distance. Ms. White was in distress and conveyed a need for help and nurturing, but it was countered by her need to distance herself for fear of expressing her anger, which resulted in her feeling deprived, frustrated, and even more needy and fearful.

The psychologist thought the patient had a strong potential for negative therapeutic reaction, with suicide being the culmination of her efforts to defeat the therapist as an expression of her frustration and rage. He also felt that, given her vulnerability to these emotional disturbances and her potential loss of impulse control with the erosion of reality testing, she might from time to time require considerable support to maintain a reflective stance, perhaps with the necessity for antidepressants.

The diagnosis of borderline personality disorder was further substantiated by the ratings of the research group on the DSM-III-R (American Psychiatric Association 1987) criteria. They reached a consensus that the patient fulfilled five criteria (unstable relationships, affective instability, inappropriate anger, identity disturbance, and chronic emptiness). A videotaped Diagnostic Interview for Borderline Patients (DIB) (Gunderson et al. 1981) was also used, and an average of the team's ratings was 5.4, which did not quite fulfill the Gunderson et al. criteria for the borderline diagnosis.

Overall, Ms. White brought to treatment a certain tenacity, buttressed by a resolute self-sufficiency. She might feel helpless in the face of overwhelming feelings of anger and subsequent spiraling depression, fearing that once the cycle had begun, things would go downhill with no turning back. Nonetheless, while anticipating that cycle and dreading it, she could say, "I have to claw myself back to the top, kick myself in the behind, tell myself to get out of it."

Predictions

Two senior clinical judges were asked to assess the patient and to predict the optimal balance between expressive versus supportive treatment techniques. They used the initial data described in Chapter 2 (this volume) in making their assessments and had no knowledge of the course of treatment. The following is a summary of their consensus judgments.

The judges anticipated that the major issue in treatment would be the patient's considerable difficulty in establishing and maintaining benign close relationships. They viewed fluctuations in closeness and distance as the "hallmark of her relatedness to others." Although hungry for emotional relatedness, once attained, she needed to reestablish a safe distance and effectively maintain "empty" relationships covered with a facade of "niceness." Further, they expected considerable work to be needed with her narcissistic vulnerability. This vulnerability led her to equate her own need for closeness with evidence of weakness, failure, and pathology. Additionally, narcissistic vulnerability evoked envious resentment when she experienced others giving to or caring for her in a manner that she could not reciprocate. The corollary of Ms. White's somewhat grandiose need to feel superior by caring for others was also viewed as a focus for work in the treatment. Still another focus was expected to be the patient's harsh and punitive superego, which induced guilt over obtaining what she wanted, heightened her fear of loss, and at times could overwhelm her ego resources.

The judges recommended a largely expressive treatment approach to deal with the "cool, distant, as if-ness of her nice persona" and to help her link the persona to her awareness of being conflicted over dimly recognized affects. There were two major exceptions identified: More supportive techniques would be needed early in the therapy and also when intense affect overwhelmed her ego resources. This might especially be the case with the emergence of intense suicidal urges and might even need to include hospitalization. For the most part, however, the judges recommended that the use of empathy should be in the form of accurate interpretations and assistance in identifying her emotional states; affirmation should be in the form of the therapist adopting a "more active and structuring presence."

The preceding predictions and recommendations were made after consideration of the following patient characteristics:

■ Ability to form an alliance, including the capacity to discuss how the emotional intensity of therapy affects her without serious acting out.

■ Conscious awareness of internal inconsistency and of a need to distance, along with concern and anxiety about these characteristics.

- Motivation to explore, change, and better herself.
- Psychological-mindedness.
- Above-average intelligence and verbal skills.

Course of Therapy

Ms. White began supportive-expressive outpatient psychotherapy immediately following a series of three interviews with an intake consultant. She was seen for a total of 143 sessions over a nearly 2-year period. The frequency of the sessions was twice a week until shortly before termination, when it was decreased to once a week.

At an appropriate interval following the initial sessions, the therapist introduced the possibility of participation in the research project. The patient gave her consent, and after the fifth session, all sessions were audiotaped. The patient agreed to participate in part because it assured her that her therapist would be attentive and do his best job.

The beginning phase of the psychotherapy was marked by the patient's acute emotional turmoil. She was in a state of severe depression, constantly preoccupied with thoughts of suicide, and absorbed in the death of her sister, whom she had been unable to mourn. The sister's death had clearly resulted in a significant disruption of the patient's nuclear family. The patient was quickly able, however, to establish a meaningful therapeutic relationship, and revealed a significant degree of reflectiveness and resilience in both her personal and professional lives. In addition to working as a social worker at an area nursing home, she also was pursuing postgraduate work leading to a master's degree in social work.

During the early sessions, Ms. White engaged in considerable self-reproach. She blamed herself in particular for her failure to recognize the multiple indications of her sister's increasing distress and the evidence of her suicidality. Her turmoil reached a crescendo as the anniversary of the sister's death approached, which subsequently subsided as she came to recognize that there were problems and issues in her own life, quite distinct from those of her sister's, that she needed to address.

As Ms. White engaged in the therapeutic work, she attempted to remain logical and organized. She also revealed hyperalertness to those moments when her therapist might not be attuned to her or be as sensitive or empathic as she wished. She mildly chastised and joked with him about his lack of responsiveness or his disengagement. Any therapist disengagement was reminiscent to her of her father's cool detachment. Ms. White also feared that her therapist would become too involved, too supportive, or too controlling in a fashion similar to her mother. Thus, she maintained a rigid but painful self-reliance that isolated her and led her to intense feelings of deprivation. Gradually she began to unveil her feelings of attachment and involvement that had both a preoedipal and an erotic character. The therapeutic work in this early phase was largely devoted to an effort to help the patient understand these transference themes.

Accompanied by much pain, fear, and occasional hatred, the patient deepened her attachment. With determination, Ms. White tried to explore experiences in the therapeutic process that reflected and repeated painful and despair-inducing experiences with her father and sister. As she stripped away some of the narcissistic self-sufficiency and allowed herself to become more dependent on the treatment process, she felt more vulnerable and frightened. She was acutely aware of her attachment and was concerned about her stability, fearing that she would lose her ability to function on the job as well as in her responsibilities at home as mother and wife.

Approximately 6 months into the therapy, the expectations of the predictors about the need for more supportive measures under the pressure of intense emotional turmoil were confirmed. The patient's concerns reached a crescendo, and she requested antidepressant medications in a rather complicated way—through her husband who became a spokesman for her difficult-to-articulate rage at her therapist/father. Ms. White's husband was concerned about the patient's severe depressive symptoms manifested by episodes of crying and obsessive suicidal thoughts. He contacted the staff social worker who had performed the initial consultation. In turn, arrangements were made for a pharmacological consultation, which led to the patient's being placed on amoxapine once more.

The patient remained on the medication for approximately 10 months before discontinuing its use. The staff social worker remained available to Ms. White's husband and saw him occasionally on an as-needed basis regarding his concerns about his wife's behavior and the course of treatment. The psychiatrist managing the medication also met with the couple on one or two occasions during periods of symptom exacerbation. These contacts were quite supportive to the psychotherapy process, as was the careful management of the medication itself.

After starting the antidepressant medication, Ms. White began to recognize the multiple and conflicted motivations associated with her request for medication and the nature of the pain that prompted it. She recognized that it was not sufficient to address those issues through medication, but rather that she needed to explore further the motivations, fantasies, and emotions associated with her request. As this work progressed, she realized that her therapist was not available to her in all the ways that she wished. Episodically, Ms. White found herself frightened and angry at the perception that the psychotherapy was hurting and injuring her as she projected her anger onto the therapist. As these issues became focused and clarified, she began to experience some relief and found renewed energy to pursue the treatment process. The patient then began to view the psychotherapist as an ally and a friend. This development was supported in part by her wish to please and to perform for the therapist as she had done at one time for her father. She was acutely aware that the psychotherapy process was taking place within a research context, and she derived some satisfaction from the knowledge that what she and her therapist did would be studied by others.

Further along in the psychotherapy, Ms. White became more acutely depressed. She tried periodically to decrease and then discontinue her antidepressant medication, only to find herself unable to do so. The patient found she was angrily turning aside her husband's overtures for sexual intimacy. She discontinued her academic pursuits and found the responsibilities of motherhood overwhelming. She became increasingly dissatisfied with the results of the psychotherapy, but it was increasingly difficult for her to communicate and to explore her internal states. She waited silently and angrily.

As the therapist attempted to probe and clarify what he understood to be the issues that most troubled her, Ms. White would nod her assent, begin to weep, and slowly expand on those issues and themes by herself. She felt extremely vulnerable, however, when accepting and utilizing help. Inevitably Ms. White found relief and understanding in the sessions; however, those improvements were followed by symptomatic worsening. For example, angry interactions with relatives occurred, problems with work appeared, and her eating disorder became exacerbated. In each instance, the increasing attachment and longing for intimacy with the therapist appeared to be the underlying dynamic that led to regressions. The patient was extremely sensitive to the rejections that were implicit in the limitations of the professional relationship, but she was loathe to express and expand on the longings that she experienced in the process. She thought that the attachment to her therapist endangered her. Her precarious state made the timing and announcement of his upcoming vacations especially problematic, given the anticipated reaction to those separations. Here the predictors' concerns about Ms. White's ability to maintain a benign relationship in the face of her narcissistic vulnerability and expectations of loss became more consistently relevant.

Ms. White became immersed in emotional turmoil in anticipation of the therapist's vacation just past midway in the therapy. The therapy sessions were marked both before and following the therapist's absence by periods of angry silence and repeated requests to reduce the frequency of the sessions from twice a week to once a week. The patient often implied, if not directly stated, that she wished not only to reduce the frequency of the sessions but to terminate. She wanted to end the pain that she thought the therapy was imposing on her. Although the patient would typically begin a session by saying that she did not want to talk and that it was too painful, more often than not she would find herself, almost against her will, beginning to experience and explore the therapeutic work more deeply. She never appeared to lose her capacity to reflect.

For example, in the first session after the therapist's return from vacation, the patient reported a significant prolonged argument with her husband, the repercussions of which persisted for several days. As Ms. White described that event, she became more animated, and with increasing delight, she detailed the satisfaction of her vengeful wishes as she attacked her husband. She said that she wanted "blood." Then reflecting on the satisfaction in her spiteful behavior, she recognized the displacement of her anger about her intense dependent needs from the therapist/father and reported that her husband recognized it as well. He had told her, in effect, "I am sick of taking this shit for your therapist and for your father." As the exploration of her anger and

vengefulness deepened, Ms. White became further aware of her increasing delight in her aggression as well as her inability to stop her
behavior. Subsequently, the patient began to explore the relationship
of these events to her underlying experience of loss and depression.

This vignette captures the centrality of the patient's struggle with
dependence and loss in the therapy. It also illustrates the limitations
of her ability to contain the intense affect stirred by these and related
transference themes. On the one hand, there was increasing evidence
of her readiness to tolerate transference intensification and to observe
and reflect on what it revealed in the psychotherapy, as well as in
outside relationships. On the other hand, there was her need to project
and disavow the sources of her pain, coupled with her wish to flee and
to restore a sense of self-sufficiency and control. A critical element
in this development was the patient's awareness that she had the power
to regulate the therapeutic process by determining the frequency of
the sessions—in essence, to flee or to triumph over her conflicts.

In the process of playing out issues of control with her husband
and the therapist, questions about finances came into focus. The staff
social worker reported that the husband would terminate the patient's
psychotherapy because of his intense dissatisfaction with his wife and
her hostile, negativistic behavior with him if we took too firm a stance
regarding fee arrangements. It became necessary to negotiate a more
extended payment plan for the patient's psychotherapy fee.

In the next phase of the treatment, the overall trend was that of
consolidation but in the context of flight from emotional pain and the
treatment process. On all fronts—in her marriage, her relationships
with her children and with colleagues at work, and her involvement
with school—Ms. White reported improved functioning and confidence. These developments took place in the context of her efforts to
move as rapidly as possible beyond her significant depressive issues.
The patient's positive relationship with the therapist deepened, and
she was increasingly responsive to transference-focused interventions, but she sought to avoid the reemergence of affect-laden, negative
transference issues. She approached the work of treatment in a vigor-
ous enough way, but ever present was the implication that she wished
to disengage, to seal over, and to reconstitute into what she called her
"perfect" state. This was the state in which the patient felt oblivious
to her rage, depression, sexual excitement, and intense longings for

an anaclitic attachment. It was a frozen emotional state in which she was impervious to the onslaught of these feelings and wishes. In that state she could be primarily an effective caretaker who would provide for others, and only reluctantly admit to herself that she wished for that which she gave to others. Associated with this effort to seal over her longings was a strong wish to compete with her husband, fellow professionals, co-workers, and therapist.

In the termination phase, the primary issue that emerged was the patient's struggle over feeling gratitude. To feel grateful and to acknowledge appreciation directly to the therapist brought with it conflicted romantic longings and the threat of giving up or changing a number of important attachments—to father, mother, siblings, children, and husband. It meant facing and renouncing the fantasy that she was indeed that special child in the family who was the center of attention, the source of strength, the source of father's resilience in his own depressive moods, and the caretaker and healer for all. In the ending phase, tender and affectionate feelings came to be expressed most directly in the therapeutic relationship. In doing so, Ms. White had to face renunciation, but she discovered a renewed interest in her husband as a sexual partner and a source of gratification of her needs for intimacy.

Part of the termination process also involved a repeated exploration of her sense of vulnerability in facing separation. We revisited her wish to seal over, function perfectly, deny her vulnerability, and ward off attachments to others who were an important source of support for her. However, this work did not alter the patient's course toward an early termination. Ms. White often used counterdependence by pressing for a reduction in the frequency of the sessions, and in fact, the frequency was reduced to once a week during the latter part of treatment. The reduction appeared to reassure the patient that she had control over the intensity of the process, which continued in this manner to an agreed-on termination date.

Assessment of Outcome

Changes in Ms. White were assessed by two clinical judges who examined the initial and termination data to evaluate the patient's changes approximately 5 years after termination of therapy. The judges believed that Ms. White had made some enduring changes.

Change was particularly notable in a better-integrated sense of self in which she felt more secure in having received nurturance and in an identity as a competent and autonomous woman who could function efficiently in her career. She had developed a more benign superego in which the previous masochistic management of her anger, her inability to accept good things, and her martyr-like display of suffering had abated. Remaining conflicts had been tempered by more adaptive defenses.

Nevertheless, the judges found that to some degree Ms. White had opted for a premature resolution of her basic conflicts, which continued albeit to a lesser degree. This premature closure was likely due to a fear of further experiencing transference dilemmas with feelings of being helpless, needy, envious, and angry. Although her defenses were more adaptive, they involved denial and projection, unstable manic and compulsive defenses, as well as idealization and heightened identification with her therapist as a good caregiver. To maintain her defensive equilibrium, Ms. White was less interested in psychological self-examination, and in that sense she was less psychologically minded and insightful than at the start of psychotherapy.

Change was substantiated by an improvement in the consensus rating on the Global Assessment Scale from an initial score of 51 (moderate symptoms or moderate difficulties in several areas) to a score of 69 (some mild symptoms or some difficulties in several areas) at follow-up. There was improvement in nearly all areas of the Bellak Scales of Ego Functions (Bellak and Goldsmith 1973) (see Appendix D, Table D–12). The Level of Functioning Scale developed by Waldinger and Gunderson (1987) also reflected improvement, particularly in the area of sense of self and, to a lesser degree, in behavior (see Appendix D, Table D–9). Finally, positive change was reflected in the DIB. The consensus score from the initial rating was 5.4, whereas the consensus score at outcome was 2.1. (a score of 7 indicates definite borderline, a score of 5 indicates "probable" borderline, and a score of 2 is well within the neurotic range).

More specifically, changes in Ms. White's internal experience and behavior were noted by the clinical judges in the following areas:

■ The patient's struggles with dependency, envy, and greed, as well as her struggle to contain resulting anger and resentment, were reduced. These conflicts were mediated by her increased stability bolstered by intensified self-sufficiency with a marked reduction in both her masochism and inability to accept what is offered to her. Those changes were noted to be enduring, freeing her to enjoy a more productive, albeit somewhat restricted and compulsive life.

■ The treatment process enabled the patient to experience a nurturing relationship that sustained her. Ms. White felt more secure in her sense of self as competent and autonomous, thereby more able to function efficiently at her work. In a parallel way, the satisfaction led to a reduction of her demands, thereby diminishing her guilt and depression. She enjoyed a more positive view of herself and an optimistic mood, maintained in part through manic and compulsive defenses. Her role as caretaker now served her wishes to display herself and her pride in her self-sufficiency, rather than as a reaction formation against her rage. Thus, the split that previously existed between a view of herself as a strong and benevolent caretaker and an abused and deprived child had been overcome to an important degree.

■ Her improved sense of well-being and the partial resolution of her internal struggles led her to devote less attention to her remaining symptoms and character problems, while paying greater attention to the real and pragmatic concerns in her life. This shift was supported by a greater reliance on denial and isolation of affect, as well as an improved self-concept.

■ The patient was less preoccupied with herself and her pain, with diminished interest in self-examination. Her reflectiveness had been displaced by the fantasy of an idealized bond with her therapist, which contributed to enhanced self-esteem and confidence in her professional competence and productiveness, characterized in part by an elevated sense of superiority.

■ Through identification with her idealized therapist, Ms. White was able to strengthen her view of herself as caretaker, thus diminishing and counterbalancing her sense of herself as angry, envious, and needing to engage in reparation for spoiling or rejecting that which was offered to her. This transformation of self-experience was bolstered in part by more effective suppression of her anger and envy, enabling her to preserve a view of herself as caretaker.

Effects of Interventions on Collaboration

The therapist's interventions and changes in the therapeutic alliance were each rated by subgroups of our research team. Consensus judgments were then reached by the entire research team about the relationship between the interventions and shifts (see Appendix A, chapter note 6).

The majority of the shifts rated in the treatment alliance (81%) were found by the raters to be linked to therapist interventions (see Appendix D, Table D–11). Although occasional key interventions immediately preceded a shift, it was striking that more often than not those pivotal interventions took place in the context of a series of interventions that had a cumulative effect and facilitated the therapeutic process. The therapeutic climate established by the therapist's attunement to the patient's emotional state appeared to be most important in providing a context that fostered the therapeutic work. On several occasions, shifts in the alliance appeared to have occurred spontaneously, without any link to particular interventions. These shifts seemed to be a product of the internal state of the patient at the time, sometimes influenced by the general climate of the therapeutic relationship.

Of the shifts that could be linked to the therapist's interventions, 76% were in the direction of an improved alliance, and 81% of these were linked to interventions that focused on the transference relationship. It was interesting to note that not only did transference-related interventions clearly lead to positive shifts in the treatment alliance, but they could also lead to negative shifts. Of the negative shifts in the alliance that could be related to therapist interventions, 80% were transference related. The interventions linked to negative shifts reflected either lack of attunement with the patient's emotional state or else fostered more intense affect than the patient was able to tolerate at the moment (see Appendix D, Table D–11).

The following is an example of a positive shift in patient collaboration that was influenced by therapist interventions related to the transference. It also vividly illustrates several aspects of the patient's conflicts with dependency, which she struggled with throughout the treatment process. The vignette comes from the session 6—the first session recorded for the research. After some discussion of the meaning of the research to her, Ms. White focuses on her wish to achieve and be perfect, in contrast to painful feelings of resentment and worthlessness, particularly in relationship to her husband.

Pt: I . . . I use a word for him that describes him so well as righteous. He's from a very staunch, Midwestern family, and that just burns me up. The righteousness about him. And so much in contrast to my family, it's *my* background. I don't see anything righteous about my background or the way our family was. It was very spontaneous and . . . like I said before . . . nonpurposeful. He's so damn righteous. [sniff] So I can see I resent him . . . at the same time. . . . [8-second pause] [unclear words] When I first met him I loved his family. I, you know, I thought his parents were great and . . . now it doesn't take much for them to irritate me. [small laugh] I even resent people at work.

Tx: Because?

Pt: I don't think they're doing a good job. I think I'm doing a better job and doing all the work sometimes. Industrious me, keeping it all together. If it wasn't for me, it would all fall apart. [laughs] That's what I start thinking.

Tx: I suspect there may be times when you feel like that with me, too.

Pt: I don't understand.

Tx: That you will feel and perhaps even now feel that you have to do all the work, carry the burden. You've been through all those painful experiences . . . and I listen . . . and I haven't shared that life with you . . . and I may seem righteous to you at times.

Pt: Very much so 'cause . . . that's the position I'm in, I think. I'm trying very hard to . . . keep myself close to your status . . . using clinical words or [sniff] large words or descriptions of things.

Tx: You can't be yourself.

Pt: [sniffs] I don't know where myself is. [tearful] I just talk 'cause you don't talk. [laughing and crying simultaneously]

Tx: Uh-huh.

Pt: I just say things that come into my head, that's all. Every time you say something it seems to . . . be right on, right on the point. It always seems to make me cry. [sniff] Did you notice that? [small laugh]

Tx: Why do you suppose that happens?

Pt: [crying] You seem to understand . . . or care. I don't know [sigh] . . . the way I see myself. [sniff] I don't ever remember being cared for in my life . . . or nurtured . . . or watched over. I'm sure I was in my very young years. I don't remember, as far as I can remember, any guidance even in my adolescence [sniff] or closeness. It's very difficult for me to feel loved, to think someone actually loves me.

The judges noted a definite positive shift ("upward shift" noted in the vignette) as the patient became more in touch with her strong feelings and was able to reflect and address them in the relationship with the therapist. The therapist's immediately preceding intervention was thought to have facilitated the shift by helping the patient establish the link between her experience in relationship to her husband and the here and now of the therapy. The therapist's intervention was considered timely, accurate, and empathic. It was actually an elaboration of an intervention that the therapist had begun two lines before. It was noted, too, that there had been considerable preparatory work that contributed to the effectiveness of this intervention. Particularly, prior interventions reflected good attunement to what the patient was attempting to communicate about her emotional state and her relationships, thereby encouraging her to elaborate.

Interestingly, the patient began the next session reporting at length about her success in writing a paper related to her work, which was well received. In so doing, she took distance from the painful feelings that she had dealt with in the previous session and attempted to reestablish herself as a professional and peer of the therapist. Similar phenomena occurred regularly during the course of therapy and were a significant characteristic in the termination phase.

Another vignette from session 89 illustrates a negative shift in patient collaboration related to transference interventions by the therapist. The vignette also illustrates how the negative shift was brought into play by the intensity of the patient's conflicts. Ms. White began the session reporting a painful argument with her husband, a sequel to an earlier argument in which he had expressed concern about her preoccupation with food and her binge eating. He also expressed concern about her progress in therapy. The vignette begins with the patient describing the escalation of the most recent argument, immediately precipitated by a perceived slight by her husband.

Pt: I said to him, "You want to bring up last night again, is that it? You want to remind me about my behavior last night? I was simply in a bad mood and tired, that's what, why I got angry at you. Can't I be in a bad mood . . . I'm not sick and you're trying to make me sick." And he said, "No, that's not what I meant," but it was all over then. It went downhill from there . . . so I had this hysterical reaction when he left me . . . now doesn't that all sound so stupid? How can I let him have so much power? I think it has something to do with being rejected by my father . . . all my life . . . and I just can't stand it from him . . . and I don't believe he loves me and I'm constantly testing him . . . that's what I think [almost in tears] . . . I guess you know the good thing about it is that we did make up and I don't feel as bad today . . . I don't feel great, but I don't feel bad . . . I didn't stay down in the depression . . . I'm so tired of all this . . . [sobbing] I don't think it's fair that he should have so much power . . . to hurt me like that . . . [sniffling sobs] . . . and I want you to make me understand it's a little . . . it'll go away and be better . . .

Tx: I'm wondering though . . . if you are . . . I'm not worried about that . . . I have a sense that the resentment you feel toward your husband for having that much power to hurt you is also a resentment you feel for *me*. At the same time you want me to have that kind of thought and interest in you. And so it would be a helpful lesson for you, if I did have that kind of power.

Pt: Like I . . . I want my husband to make things better sometimes . . . you know . . . it's the same thing . . . it's like I wanted him to talk to me about my eating, my obsession. I want him to make them better . . . [tearful voice] I want you to make things better . . . I see that problem with my husband, I see . . . an enormous one . . . it causes me great pain. [long pause]

Tx: What are you thinking?

[down- *Pt:* I'm thinking about work . . . well, I don't feel as well today . . .
ward   I . . . I wonder how I'm going to feel there? . . . when I don't feel
shift]   as well . . . I'm feeling like . . . you're leaving it up to me to get
              well . . . to get better over this problem and I've got . . . don't feel
              able to do that . . . [tearful]

The judges noted a probable downward shift when Ms. White said, "I'm thinking about work." The therapist had previously invited the patient to consider that her anger over her husband's apparent power to hurt her might also be present in the treatment relationship. The patient rejected the intervention and changed the subject, moved away from the transference, and then responded as if the therapist had abandoned her. Although the therapist's intervention was seen as reasonably accurate, it was not particularly well timed and appeared to lack adequate attunement to the intensity of the patient's emotions and defensive needs. For the moment at least, the patient could not accept dealing with the issue of the therapist's power. Ms. White needed to keep her own feelings of powerlessness and anger directed at the external persecutor, her husband, with herself as the victim. Correspondingly, she wanted to maintain a benign relationship with the therapist in which he would magically cure and rescue her while she maintained the stance of helplessness and inadequacy. This characteristically borderline object relations split was not amenable to further therapeutic work at this point.

A final brief vignette also serves to illustrate the importance of empathic attunement to this patient in the treatment process and the effect of more supportive interventions when needed. The vignette comes from two sessions later: session 91. The patient began by reporting feeling depressed and anxious, with concern about her ability to function adequately. She had binged since the last session and now introduces the thought that she might benefit from an eating disorder group. After tracking the patient closely for some time, the therapist provides the patient with a summary of his understanding of the conflicts she is struggling with, including the temptation for her to give up and the wish for him to take over. The interventions are more lengthy than usual and are geared to encourage and support her adaptive ability, as well as to explain. The vignette begins after a long silence, during which the patient apparently reflects on what the therapist has said thus far.

Pt: I feel caught in the middle. Therapy's supposed to be helpful, yet it . . . doesn't fulfill the vast needs that I have. I get disappointed. I don't feel strong enough to deal with it on my own. I really feel like a mess today. [sniff]

Tx: Here's another . . . and this is a point that I have made, I think I've made before that there's another side to it, too, and, uh, um . . . for the first time as far as I know of you've tried to . . . bring these things into focus without being perfect . . . and without running away from it . . . I think you experience these things in some way as, uh, [unclear words] I can't recall exactly the word you used, uh, to talk about what it would be like in with the group.

Pt: Another stigma . . .

Tx: Stigma.

Pt: To deal with. I feel like I'm getting lower and lower on the, on the . . . [sigh, small laugh]

Tx: Scale.

Pt: Scale of humanity.

Tx: Well . . . maybe I'm being Pollyannish in saying this . . . um, I think you're trying to face things in yourself and your life, um, more directly and more intensely than you have before. I don't see it entirely as such a [unclear words].

Pt: It makes me cry almost out of happiness to think when you said I'm facing things more directly and I had that thought when I started . . . realizing I was thinking about the eating disorder group, I thought . . . I wonder if that's a *good* sign instead of a bad sign. And when you said that I . . . I almost started crying again . . . because, um, because of the . . . maybe the thought that I'm not as bad as I thought I was or as bad as I feel like I am today. It's painful to look at all these things about myself.

The judges noted a definite positive shift when Ms. White said, "It makes me cry. . . ." The basis for the judgment was the patient's expression of feeling helped, increased expression of affect, and increased collaboration with the therapist in making use of his interventions. The interventions in this vignette were most clearly linked to fostering the shift in collaboration, providing affirmation that helped the patient feel acknowledged for her efforts and value. These interventions and those that preceded provided the patient with partial gratification of her transference wishes while still managing to bolster her self-esteem. Equally significant, the therapist avoided directly addressing Ms. White's hints of continued dissatisfaction with him, including those implicit in the consideration of other forms of treatment.

The therapist's shift from a more characteristic interpretive approach at this point appeared to be determined by several factors. Ms. White was in the midst of a regression that the therapist believed required more support and containment. She had recently discontinued antidepressant medication, which contributed to the regression and the need to provide additional support. As observed in the previous vignette from two sessions earlier, a transference-focused interpretive approach was not effective under the circumstances, leaving the patient feeling that the therapist was out of tune with her needs and distant or uncaring.

The ratings of the judges for this case indicate considerable consistency in the use of different types of interventions and in the use of transference-focused interventions over the course of treatment. Likewise, a clear pattern regarding changes in collaboration also emerged from the data. Although the overall level of collaboration did not differ noticeably at the end of therapy in comparison with the beginning, there were significant differences between the beginning and the end of each session. Of the 18 sessions rated, 12 registered a higher collaboration rating during the last third of the session than during the first third. Only one session was judged to have a lower level of collaboration at the end than at the beginning.

Discussion

In our discussion of the process and outcome of Ms. White's psychotherapy, we focus on patient factors that contributed to her suitability
for a modified exploratory approach and on aspects of therapeutic
strategy and style responsive to those factors. Prior to that discussion,
we need to address the question of diagnosis.

Diagnosis

In view of Ms. White's professional achievements and compliant "as-
if" character style, one could question whether she fit within the
spectrum of borderline disorders. At the beginning of treatment, the
patient was in the midst of an acute depressive suicidal crisis, a state
of prolonged emotional anguish precipitated by the suicide of her
sister 2 years prior to seeking treatment. She was also a member of a
severely dysfunctional family. Her siblings were chronically troubled, were suicidal, and had significant characterological problems.
For 5 years before the beginning of treatment, the patient had been
bulimic and unresponsive to a course of antidepressant medication.
Her emotional turbulence, depressive suicidal state, bulimia, en-
meshment in a dysfunctional family, and chronic low self-esteem led
the referring consultant to the diagnostic conclusion that Ms. White
was functioning in the borderline range. This finding was confirmed by
the emergence of primary process thinking on the psychological tests.

The testing additionally revealed identity diffusion, prominent
masochistic features, vulnerability to affective flooding and dyscontrol, developmental disturbances at the separation-individuation
phase, potential for psychotic regression, and great problems in regulating interpersonal distance (oscillating between detachment and regressive overinvolvement). The psychological test report also
emphasized the patient's underlying rage and potential for negative
therapeutic reaction, including suicide. These vulnerabilities led to
the prediction that she would perhaps require considerable support
and most likely a resumption of the antidepressant medication.

Finally, significant characterological difficulties were noted in the
testing, manifest most clearly in the narcissistic and compulsive features that led to her excessive concern with appearance and the tendency to distance herself from others with a rigid investment in work.

We thus concluded that diagnostically Ms. White fell in the middle to upper end of the borderline range. We are in accord with Meissner (1984) that the borderline diagnosis encompasses a spectrum of characterological disturbance and ego weakness ranging from those who are overtly psychotic to those who function close to the neurotic range. Those at the upper reaches of the borderline spectrum are considered to be more amenable to an exploratory, uncovering, reconstructive approach (Abend et al. 1983). The follow-up consensus rating on the DIB reflected an overall treatment improvement moving from an initial rating of 5.4 to 2.1. The structural change implied in such a shift indicated to us that the patient was functioning at termination within the neurotic range.

Developmental Factors

The patient's history revealed no evidence of discrete, early trauma. Rather, there was evidence of prolonged, uninterrupted exposure to chronic marital turmoil in a dysfunctional family that left her as the parentified child inappropriately responsible for the emotional well-being of her mother, father, and siblings. For example, Ms. White had vivid memories of confronting her father at moments of imminent physical violence, staring him down while protecting her mother from physical injury. She learned repeatedly from an early age to mute awareness and expression of age-appropriate childhood needs. She was instead recruited to assume the role of caretaker, leading to the development of a false self. As Pine (1990) noted, developmental deficiencies—that is, the absence of or significant distortion of parental functions—can result in developmentally based deficits in ego functioning. The development of her self-sufficiency; narcissistic character defenses; unresolved grandiosity; vulnerability to shame, rage, envy, and so on can be understood in this context. This paradigm as the self-sufficient caretaker served as the nucleus for her pattern of stifling emergent transference wishes in the psychotherapy.

Ego Factors

Motivation for change.　The patient's acute emotional turbulence at the beginning of the treatment process, characterized by a suicidal depressive crisis and bulimia, frightened the patient sufficiently and served as a powerful impetus to initiate a treatment process sustained by additional powerful motivations: the wish to abate profound feelings of guilt, alleviate painful feelings of shame and inferiority, redress a deteriorating marital relationship, resume important professional goals, bolster a flagging sense of self-mastery and self-sufficiency, and come to terms with disparate and contradictory versions of herself. Most broadly, she sought to achieve changes in her character and behavior to permit her to function effectively.

Capacity to work in an analytic space. Ms. White's capacity to enter into the shadow theater of the mind and to engage the therapist playfully as though he were a version of figures from her childhood and adolescence was variable. Given her developmental deficiencies, she sought a "real" relationship that would make up for what she had found missing. Thus, therapeutic abstinence and neutrality proved frustrating; warmth and implicit mirroring were welcomed responses to her developmental needs. Granted the pressure for transference gratification, the patient was open, but painfully so, to transference explorations. In a limited and focused way, she was able to give voice to the link between transference frustrations and antecedent deficiencies in her relationship with parents.

Impulse control and affect tolerance. Although characterologically disposed to detachment and reserve, Ms. White was capable of considerable warmth and tolerance of dysphoric states. Although her warmth facilitated a close therapeutic collaboration, and her tolerance of dysphoric states made circumscribed explorations of emotionally turbulent issues possible, the patient had important limits. In particular, protracted states of intense rage and envy became progressively unmanageable, leading to displacement and acting out in her marital relationship; episodic bulimia; and, presented in its more extreme form, a risk crucial to the stability and continuity of the psychotherapy. The psychological tests had underscored her potential for suicide, negative therapeutic reaction, and psychotic regression in the face of severely taxing emotional experiences. Thus, titrating the intensity of her transference experiences was required to help the patient moderate surges of what might be intensely destabilizing emotional storms. As is described later, a number of specific factors related to the style of addressing the negative transference, responding to emotional crisis, and moderating the intensity of the transference relationship were called into play as a result of this core vulnerability.

Proneness to externalization. Projective blaming of Ms. White's husband became a central theme of the psychotherapy process. From early in their marriage, he had served a number of selfobject functions. He provided economic and emotional stability while serving as a container for her rage, as well as a moderator of her excesses and a resource to stave off loneliness. Before and during much of Ms. White's psychotherapy, he became the target for her displaced aggression. At one point, he protested that he was no longer going to take her "shit" for her therapist and father. His rigidity oppressed her, and his plainness and lack of excitement stifled her sexually. He shamed her and made her feel selfish and guilty. He was both her persecutor and repository of disowned aspects of herself. Primarily, the patient's husband was the target of incessant projective identification (Lachkar 1992). Over the course of the therapy, she gradually was able to confront her pattern of displaced and acted-out frustration and aggression and its sources in her relationship with her father, thus surrendering some of the externalization and projective identification. That resolution led to an improved marital relationship. Her developing capacity over the course of the psychotherapy to confront, clarify, and examine this pattern of externalization contributed to her improved therapeutic alliance and treatment outcome.

Psychological-mindedness. Ms. White had a fascination with understanding the underlying emotional states of her family members, colleagues, and patients, taking great pride in her capacity to come to terms with the complex interplay of competing motivations arising in the patient-treater relationship. She was both shamed and fascinated by that prospect in the psychotherapy and demonstrated a persistent interest in unearthing and confronting her own motivations.

Relationship Factors

Narcissistic vulnerability. Ms. White's narcissistic vulnerability was considerable and rooted in several factors: her shame propensity, grandiosity, and guilt. The emergence and discovery of transference wishes inevitably provoked experiences of embarrassment; she would often blush profusely. She was furiously devoted to maintaining her self-sufficiency and to maintaining her position as the most competent caretaker in her family. She could surrender that version of herself only with great reluctance. She experienced immense guilt for her failure to correct the emotional flaws of her parents and siblings. Finally, Ms. White was troubled with the emergence of transference wishes that expressed needs for affirmation and support. The therapeutic exploration of each of these issues resulted in repeated experiences of shame and injury to her self-esteem. This cycle proved to be a major resistance to a further deepening of the therapeutic relationship and contributed to the termination of the psychotherapy.

Mirroring and idealizing transferences. Idealization as a defensive avoidance of primitive aggression and devaluation of the therapist does not appear to have played a major part in the therapeutic process. Rather, an enduring theme was the patient's search for an affirming parental relationship that would serve her developmental needs. She appeared to be frustrated with her husband's failures in attunement, sensing the absence of age-appropriate supports for her thwarted developmental achievements. Thus, an important component of the therapeutic relationship was the affirmation of those aspects of herself that she valued and wished to develop. Communicative matching appeared to be especially important for her, giving form as it did to her wish for a lively, involved, interested relatedness with her father.

Distancing and counterdependency. Consistently, the patient reasserted her self-sufficiency following the emergence of powerful transference wishes. Inevitably, her longings for contact or engagement evoked feelings of rage, shame, vulnerability, and envy, which were transferentially related to her turbulent attachments to her parents, especially her father, a distant and troubled man. The reassertion of her position as the most competent eldest child in a chaotic family, solely responsible for the emotional well-being and functioning of that family, played itself out at work, in her marriage, and in the therapeutic relationship. This conflict and its appearance in the therapeutic relationship presented the patient and her therapist with an opportunity to explore and resolve a key relational difficulty in the patient's life, which also established important limits on the extent of change possible and the style of exploring that issue.

Although the judges noted that Ms. White had made enduring changes, specifically in a better integrated sense of self, a more benign superego, and more adaptive defenses, they also observed that she had chosen to terminate therapy prematurely. The patient's motivations for terminating therapy, according to the judges, were envy, rage, intense neediness, and fear of revisiting transference regressions marked by feelings of helplessness. The judges also believed that for her to achieve and maintain her defensive equilibrium, the patient diminished her interest in psychological self-examination. Most broadly, the factor limiting the impact of the psychotherapy was her self-sufficiency. That stance had been destabilized prior to beginning treatment, was threatened by the emergence of increasingly powerful transference experiences, and was vigorously reinstated to overcome powerful feelings of shame, vulnerability, rage, and envy. Once the borderline dilemmas were addressed and resolved to some degree through the therapeutic work, the patient's narcissistic character defenses again became a prominent source of stabilization, although modified to some important degree.

Clinging and symbiotic needs. Ms. White was most shamed by the emergence of her wishes to find a protective relationship in the psychotherapy. She had fought valiantly as a child and adolescent to suppress those needs in the service of maintaining her position as the parentified child, responsible as the oldest child for the emotional safety and well-being of her siblings and parents. Thus, she was led to suppress and deny those earliest developmental wishes. There was no relationship in her professional life, family, or friendships that could be characterized as clinging or symbiotic.

Sadistic and erotized transference. Although erotic wishes emerged gradually and in disguised form, there were no indications that Ms. White engaged in an erotized relationship with her therapist. Sadistic elements in the transference were enacted in the marital relationship. Her husband appeared to be trapped in a sadomasochistic relationship, with her becoming the target for those conflicts. For example, she may well have acted out an aspect of her identification with her father by depriving her husband of sexual and emotional intimacy in a provocative fashion.

Capacity for concern. A major theme in Ms. White's life was her awareness of the impact of her aggressive assaults on others, her concern for their welfare, and the wish to make reparation while feeling guilty and responsible. She felt enormously guilty for the suicide of her sister. Despite the reality that she had been compassionate, sensitive, and supportive, she feared nonetheless that a minor slight may have precipitated her sister's suicide. More broadly, Ms. White felt trapped by the emotional vulnerability of each family member and was thus resentfully attentive to their many needs. She was able in her professional life to give less conflicted attention to her clients and, in fact, was remarkably attuned to their needs, wishes, and fantasies. Her exaggerated, guilt-laden concern for others and her wish to achieve a more realistic and balanced engagement in the lives of her husband, children, nuclear family, and professional colleagues served as an important supporting motive for her engagement in psychotherapy.

Flexibility Hypothesis

Ms. White did not comfortably enter into intimate relationships. She preferred a cool, well-controlled distance from others and permitted herself warmth and spontaneity with others in only selected relationships. Passion, warmth, and spontaneity could develop only after a cautious evaluation of the safety of a relationship rooted in carefully establishing boundaries. Thus she entered into the psychotherapy process reluctantly, permitting warmth, intimacy, and a trustful exploration of fantasies and wishes under conditions that she controlled. Inevitably, she retreated from these moments of closeness, reestablishing her self-sufficiency, while concretely controlling the frequency and length of the treatment. The therapeutic exploration of her difficulties in establishing intimate relationships yielded some gain; nonetheless, her intolerance of closeness led to premature termination.

Therapeutic Approaches

Assessing collaboration. Despite changes in the emotional climate of the relationship associated with the emergence of disturbing transference themes that altered the patient's perception of the bond with the therapist, the patient's capacity to maintain a working relationship with the therapist remained consistent throughout. With but one exception, Ms. White deepened her collaboration in each session (see Appendix A, chapter note 7).

Pattern of interventions. An exploratory uncovering of unconscious conflict and its resolution through an expressive process focused on the transference was recommended by an independent group of judges evaluating data available at the beginning of treatment. The judges also recommended that such expressive, uncovering efforts would need to be bolstered periodically by supportive parameters, such as antidepressant medication. Modifications in the balance of supportive and expressive elements were required in the face of the patient's affect intolerance.

The literature on the treatment of borderline patients in an expressive, exploratory mode has increasingly emphasized the role of supportive measures to structure and contain the emotional turbulence activated by the mobilization of more primitive transference experiences (Kernberg et al. 1989). Interestingly, in the middle phase of the treatment, a downward shift in the Luborsky Type I therapeutic alliance ratings reflected some deterioration of the patient's sense of bonding with the therapist. There was, however, a concomitant upward shift in the ratings of the supportive activity of the therapist. In addition to the within-session increase in supportive interventions, the therapist also referred the patient for pharmacotherapy (antidepressants) and marital therapy and, at one point, offered brief inpatient psychiatric hospitalization. This reflected a shift in therapeutic strategy occasioned by the therapist's efforts to respond to regressive shifts in the transference and the activation of turbulent, difficult-to-contain emotional states. Despite the increase in supportive measures, the therapist's exploratory, transference-focused efforts did not decline. In fact, the therapist engaged in a markedly increased effort to explore the patient's experience of the therapeutic relationship, as noted, for example, by the preponderance of relationship-focused interventions and encouragements to elaborate concurrent with an increased frequency of transference interpretations. Thus, the therapist used a mixed expressive-supportive strategy to address emotional crisis.

The fostering of a therapeutic alliance with a borderline patient hinges in large measure on the patient's perception that the therapist is a reliable and safe container of emotional turbulence and unrestrained action. From the beginning of the therapeutic process, the therapist sought to tolerate and metabolize Ms. White's suicidal rage and despair that were occasioned by her profound separation-abandonment experience and her overwhelming guilt associated with her sister's suicide. That first encounter served as the basis for the initial high level of the alliance.

The management of the negative transference appears also to have played an enduring role. The thwarting of transference wishes and the resultant frustration and rage were episodically and intensely enacted in the marital relationship, leading to a developing crisis requiring intervention by her pharmacotherapist and social worker. The therapist's tolerance of the splitting and displacement, while maintaining a supportive atmosphere, and his efforts to address directly the negative transference through interpretation appear to have helped the patient maintain a therapeutic relationship in the midst of this turmoil. The therapist's style was to foster elaboration of therapeutic metaphors that gave expression to those displaced affects and then to address the transference in the here and now, pointing out the patient's frustration and rage with him.

Other technical considerations. Throughout, the therapist made a concerted effort to address Ms. White's reassertion of her self-sufficiency as a transference defense. These problems were consistently explored in the here and now, while permitting disengagement and detachment. The patient's flight and its immediate sources in her emotional state (rage, anger, jealousy, envy, shame, guilt) were then explored. Left implicit and not genetically reconstructed were the broader, historical, developmental antecedents to this transference drama. Leaving to the patient the option to explore those genetic antecedents evoked by transference reenactments was a facet of the therapist's strategy to permit distance and disengagement in the context of intimacy. He thus implicitly acknowledged the patient's strong characterological disposition toward self-sufficiency, embedded in her fears of a merger transference and loss of self. The frequency of the sessions—twice a week tapered to once a week for the last phase of the treatment process—reflected such an approach as well. By reducing the number of sessions, the therapist implicitly acknowledged the patient's need for distance.

Countertransference. Countertransference manifestations were largely managed silently without direct expression in the therapeutic process, but were reflected more in the therapist's positive regard for the patient and her capacity for therapeutic work. The therapist was willing to participate and provide silently for Ms. White's mirroring and idealizing needs. This in turn may well have promoted her increasing capacity to trust the therapeutic setting so she could undergo a more intensive therapeutic regression—with both its negative and positive elements—in the service of therapeutic change. For example, she was able explicitly to express her wishes and fantasies, while clearly seeking to disengage and reestablish a position of narcissistic self-sufficiency.

Summary

Ms. White was a married, professional woman in her early 30s who had sought consultation in the midst of an increasingly difficult depressive crisis precipitated by the suicide of a younger sister 2 years earlier. The patient had been raised in a largely dysfunctional family with chronic marital discord and poor boundaries where, as the oldest sibling, she had been recruited as a family caretaker.

The nearly 2-year psychotherapy was conducted on an outpatient basis twice weekly, largely in an exploratory mode but with intermittent shifts to more supportive strategies (e.g., antidepressant medication, family therapy) occasioned by the patient's emotional turbulence. Nonetheless, the therapist maintained a focus on the transference throughout.

Two clinical judges conducted an independent assessment of the clinical outcome of the psychotherapy process and noted enduring changes, particularly in a better integrated sense of self, supported by a more benign superego and reduced masochism. Treatment limitations involved premature termination of the psychotherapy with some remaining conflicts, defensive instability, and reduced psychological-mindedness. Internalization of the idealized caregiver/therapist was believed to be an agent of change.

Several factors limited the effectiveness of the mixed expressive-supportive psychotherapy: self-sufficiency, narcissistic vulnerability, affect intolerance, externalization, transference acting out, intolerance of intimacy, diminished trust, and symptom relief. Specifically, parentification as the eldest child in a dysfunctional family led to the development of a character style in which self-sufficiency played a prominent role. Shifts in that stance led to rage, envy, shame, and, more broadly, to affective instability and the risk of disorganization. The emergence of normal developmental needs in the transference and their elaboration led to feelings of intense shame and envy. Exposure of her underlying guilt created considerable anxiety. Therapeutic exploration of those issues evoked frequent injury to her self-esteem from which she retreated—a cycle that contributed to the premature termination of the psychotherapy.

Frustration of neurotic wishes in the transference and therapeutic failures in attunement evoked rage, devaluation, and feelings of deprivation and aloneness. Provocative acting out of these affects in her marriage led to her husband's retaliations that threatened the continuity of the treatment. She only reluctantly acknowledged this pattern as a feature of the transference, because she preferred to maintain an idealizing relationship. She preferred a well-controlled distance from others, permitting warmth, spontaneity, passion, and the trustful involvement with another only under carefully controlled circumstances.

Symptom relief reduced Ms. White's motivation to continue. A powerful motive for the patient's initiation of the psychotherapy was her acute emotional turbulence and deteriorating marital relationship. The therapeutic process resolved those symptoms, leading to internal and interpersonal calm; thus, a powerful impetus to continue was removed. Additionally, she was in a reasonably stable and supportive marital relationship, albeit strained by her emotional crisis. That, plus her capacity for professional achievement, led to further stability and satisfaction in her life. Implicit was the sense that she had achieved the best adaptation possible. A more ambitious process might have threatened her achievements and her adaptations.

Five main factors contributed to Ms. White's successful participation in an exploratory approach to her difficulties: 1) her ability to form an alliance; 2) her awareness of and wish to address internal inconsistencies; 3) her motivation to explore, change, and better herself; 4) her psychological-mindedness; and 5) her intellectual and verbal talents. To a lesser degree, her relative capacity to tolerate dysphoric states and her willingness, albeit grudgingly, to enter into transference explorations contributed to some degree of examination of the transference. Also, she had a wish to redress her guilt-laden involvement in the lives of her family and to achieve a more realistic and balanced engagement with them. Paradoxically, the factor that proved to be most severely limiting regarding the continued exploration of internal conflict—that is, her self-sufficiency—proved also to be crucial to the successful resolution of the psychotherapy process and her posttreatment adjustment. Specifically, Ms. White had the pluck, determination, and courage to persevere through extraordinary emotional pain. She fiercely sought to prevail as an effective caretaker, mother, and professional. Finally, an important aspect of the idealized relationship with her therapist was her perception of his support for her survival, growth, and development as a competent adult woman.

References

Abend SM, Porder MS, Willick MS: Borderline Patients: Psychoanalytic Perspectives. New York, International Universities Press, 1983

American Psychiatric Association: Diagnostic and Statistical Manual of Mental Disorders, 3rd Edition, Revised. Washington, DC, American Psychiatric Association, 1987

Bellak L, Goldsmith L: The Broad Scope of Ego Function Assessment. New York, Wiley, 1973

Gunderson JG, Kolb JE, Austin V: The Diagnostic Interview for Borderline Patients. Am J Psychiatry 138:896–903, 1981

Kernberg OF, Selzer MA, Koenigsberg HW, et al: Psychodynamic Psychotherapy With Borderline Patients. New York, Basic Books, 1989

Lachkar J: The Narcissistic Borderline Couple: A Psychoanalytic Perspective on Marital Treatment. New York, Brunner/Mazel, 1992

Meissner WW: The Borderline Spectrum: Differential Diagnosis and Developmental Issues. New York, Jason Aronson, 1984

Pine F: Drive, Ego, Object, and Self. New York, Basic Books, 1990

Waldinger RJ, Gunderson JG: Effective Psychotherapy With Borderline Patients: Case Studies. Washington, DC, American Psychiatric Press, 1987

Tailoring the Psychotherapy to the Patient

A basic axiom of good clinical work is that the treatment must be adjusted to the patient, not the patient to the treatment. The intensive case studies in the three preceding chapters provide us with a wealth of data that allow us to propose some tentative answers to the questions raised in the introductory chapter of this volume. Our quest to define the optimal treatment for each borderline patient requires analysis of our data at several levels: 1) a construction of intervention profiles *across* sessions as well as trends in collaboration throughout the psychotherapy, 2) examination of how the therapist's interventions influence the moment-to-moment shifts in collaboration *within* individual sessions, 3) a comparison of therapist approaches and patient responses among the three psychotherapies studied, and 4) an attempt to identify patient characteristics that assist the therapist in deciding the appropriate emphasis of expressive and supportive elements in a particular therapy process with a particular patient. We also present conclusions regarding the nature of mutative factors in the psychotherapy of borderline patients. However, we first examine the variable of outcome, because a microanalysis of process is meaningless unless it is anchored to an assessment of the extent and nature of change in the patient.

143

Outcome

In each of the three cases, the independent judges assessed that significant improvement had taken place. In addition to substantial positive changes in the evaluated ego functions, the Global Assessment Scale improved from a minimum of 18 points (Ms. White) to a maximum of 30 points (Mr. Black). Also, the four levels of functioning scales were assessed before and after treatment and showed considerable improvement across the board on all three cases.

Of the three patients, only Mr. Black stayed in therapy long enough (7 years) to reach a mutual termination agreement with his therapist. Both Ms. Green and Ms. White were clearly taking flight from therapy and, from the perspectives of their therapists, were prematurely terminating. As our outcome assessments demonstrate, therapists should not be discouraged when faced with a patient who is determined to end the therapy much earlier than the therapist thinks is optimal. Substantial gains are clearly possible even from interrupted treatments. Moreover, as Gunderson (1992) noted, many borderline patients ultimately benefit from the "bucket-brigade" phenomenon of having a series of therapists over time who collectively make a cumulative impact on the patient.

Any discussion of outcome in these three cases must take into account that psychotherapy was not the only modality involved in the treatment of these patients. Mr. Black and Ms. Green spent a considerable amount of time in extended hospital treatment and later partial hospitalization. In addition to the direct effects of treatment from an array of ancillary treaters, the inpatient units and day hospital experiences provided a holding environment that allowed the psychotherapists to risk more expressive or exploratory approaches. Gunderson (1984) and Kernberg (1984) suggest that an intensive psychotherapeutic approach should not be attempted with borderline patients unless a hospital environment is available as backup to contain the patient's affective responses and impulsive discharges associated with the therapy. Mr. Black and Ms. Green also required pharmacotherapy as part of their treatment. Ms. White, although not requiring hospitalization, needed antidepressant medication, and social work assistance was needed with the patient's husband. Although we cannot attribute all the improvement in these patients to the psychotherapy alone, we must recognize that multiple treaters and treatment settings are the *rule* rather than the exception in the treatment courses of borderline patients. Moreover, our focus on a microanalysis of the process of individual sessions allows us to study the influence of the therapist's interventions on the patient under a magnifying glass.

Expressive Versus Supportive Techniques

The juxtaposition of these three psychotherapy processes creates a rich portrait of the complexities and challenges inherent in the psychotherapeutic treatment of borderline patients. In our effort to describe this portrait, we begin with the broad brush strokes before moving to the fine details of the texture. Perhaps the most global assessments made by the research team were the dimensions of expressiveness and supportiveness. Expressiveness was rated on a numerical scale from 1 to 7, with a rating of 1 signifying the least expressive and a rating of 7 reflecting the most expressive. A similar rating system was used for the supportiveness dimension. We compare these ratings across the three cases in Table 6–1.

The figures in Table 6–1 represent mean ratings for the expressive and supportive dimensions of each of the psychotherapy sessions rated. Mr. Black and Ms. White had psychotherapies that were equally expressive, but Ms. White's psychotherapy was somewhat more supportive than Mr. Black's. Ms. Green clearly had the least expressive and the most supportive psychotherapy.

Another method of evaluating the expressive-supportive dimension is by measuring the degree to which the therapist's interventions focused on the transference. In Table 6–2 we compare the extent of

Table 6–1. Expressive and supportive dimensions (mean ratings)

Patient	Expressive	Supportive
Mr. Black	5.6	2.6
Ms. Green	4.1	4.4
Ms. White	5.6	3.3

Table 6–2. Transference versus extratransference focus of interventions (mean number/session)

Patient	Transference	Extratransference
Mr. Black	10.2	10.5
Ms. Green	10.7	63.1
Ms. White	13.2	10.3

focus on transference versus extratransference issues by looking at the mean number of transference interventions and extratransference interventions per session.

The number of therapist comments that focused on the transference relationship did not vary greatly across the three cases. In the psychotherapies of Mr. Black and Ms. White, the number of extratransference interventions was roughly similar to the number of transference-focused statements by the therapists. However, in the case of Ms. Green, the therapist made six comments focused on issues outside the therapeutic relationship for every one transference intervention, again reflecting a greater degree of supportiveness than in the other two cases.

Yet a third method of assessing the expressive-supportive dimension of a psychotherapy process is by inspecting the relative weight of different therapist interventions along a continuum of the most

Table 6–3. Continuum of therapist interventions: mean number and percentage of each type of intervention per session

	Mr. Black		Ms. Green		Ms. White	
	Mean	%	Mean	%	Mean	%
Interpretation	5.2	25.1	4.2	5.7	3.3	14.1
Confrontation	2.6	12.6	18.6	25.2	5.1	21.8
Clarification	3.8	18.4	10.2	13.8	0.8	3.4
Encouragement to elaborate	8.7	42.0	35.1	47.6	12.5	53.4
Empathy	0.0	0	0.8	1.1	0.2	0.9
Advice and praise	0.4	1.9	4.9	6.6	1.6	6.8
Total	20.7		73.8		23.5	

expressive (interpretation) to the least expressive (affirmation). Table 6–3 provides an overview of the average number and percentage of each type of intervention per session in the three different processes.

The total number of interventions per session is striking in that Ms. Green's therapist used nearly 3.5 times the total number of interventions per session as the therapists treating Mr. Black and Ms. White. This increased activity level itself may be considered a reflection of a more supportive treatment. That Ms. Green's psychotherapy was much less expressive than the other two is confirmed by the lower proportion of interpretations per session (5.7% compared with Mr. Black's 25.1% and Ms. White's 14.1%). The greater use of support in Ms. Green's and Ms. White's treatments may be reflected in the higher proportion of interventions involving advice and praise.

In summary, the most expressive treatment was Mr. Black's, and the least expressive was Ms. Green's, with Ms. White's falling between the other two. The inverse is true for the supportiveness dimension.

Collaboration

Our principal measure of the impact of therapist interventions involve whether the patient's collaboration improved as a result of the intervention. In this regard, shifts in collaboration were viewed as "mini-outcomes" within the sessions. In addition, we measured broad patterns of collaboration across sessions so that we could draw profiles that characterize the patient's collaboration with the therapist throughout the course of psychotherapy. Figure 6–1 juxtaposes the mean collaboration ratings per session across each of the three psychotherapy processes.

An examination of the graphs in Figure 6–1 reveals several findings of considerable interest. First of all, although all three patients showed up and down movement during the course of psychotherapy, none of them showed dramatic improvements in collaboration as a result of psychotherapy. Both Ms. Green and Ms. White ended therapy at a somewhat lower level than they began, whereas Mr. Black collaborated with his therapist at a slightly higher level than measured at the beginning. Ms. Green averaged the lowest level of collaboration, and Ms. White was in between the two. If collaboration is viewed as

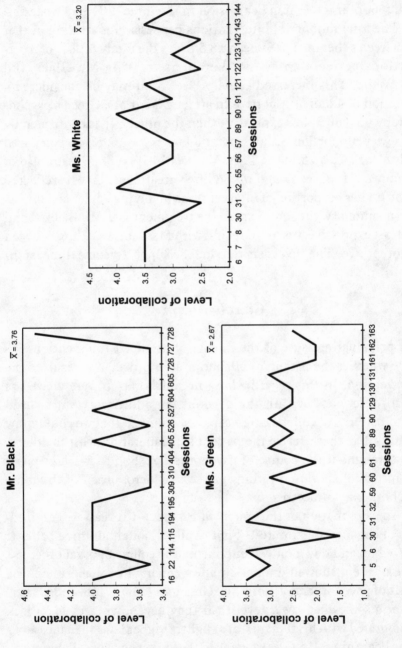

Figure 6–1. Changes in patient collaboration across sessions.

an outcome measure, our data certainly do not support the notion that borderline patients improve in a gradual stepwise manner across the course of psychotherapy.

All three patients appeared to start out with a reasonably good therapeutic alliance only to have it collapse to some extent after the treatment got going. Indeed, many borderline patients begin treatment with an idealizing transference and gradually deteriorate as inevitable frustrations make the therapist appear less than ideal. This initial idealization, followed by deterioration in the patient's ability to collaborate, is often paralleled by a feeling of optimism in the therapist, followed by a growing skepticism about the patient's ability to use treatment. Borderline patients may appear highly motivated and psychologically minded at the beginning of therapy, and their regression after a few sessions may catch the therapist off guard. Many therapists in such situations assume that this collapse is iatrogenic rather than the natural course of the condition when the patient is involved in an intense one-to-one relationship.

Figures 6–2 and 6–3 reflect ratings across sessions for all three cases on the Luborsky Type I and Type II measures of the therapeutic alliance.

As noted earlier, the Type I alliance measures the degree to which the patient experiences the therapist as warm, helpful, and supportive, whereas the Type II alliance is based on the perception that therapist and patient are working together in a joint effort to overcome what is impeding the patient. Ms. Green did not show a great deal of difference from Mr. Black and Ms. White overall in terms of the Luborsky Type I rating. However, on the Type II ratings, she came out significantly lower than Mr. Black and Ms. White consistently throughout the course of her psychotherapy.

One interpretation of the major discrepancy between Ms. Green and the other patients in the Type II rating, associated with little difference in the Type I rating, is that Ms. Green was able to experience her therapist as warm and supportive but was nevertheless unable to collaborate smoothly with him. This observation may reflect a split transference as well. Throughout most of her psychotherapy, Ms. Green was in a setting where multiple treaters were involved. She typically idealized her psychotherapist while devaluing her hospital doctor and the inpatient treatment team. Hence, the apparently good

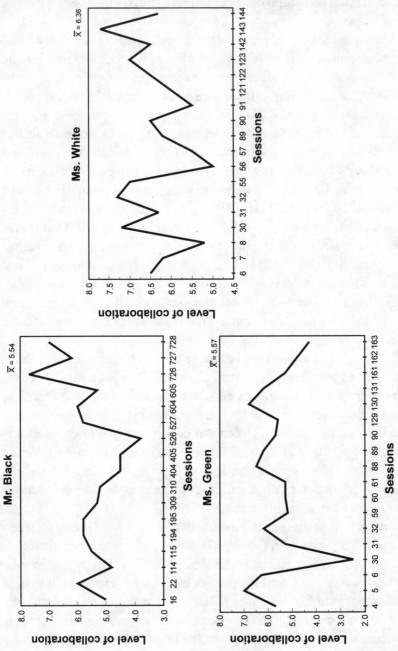

Figure 6–2.   Changes in Luborsky Type I therapeutic alliance across sessions.

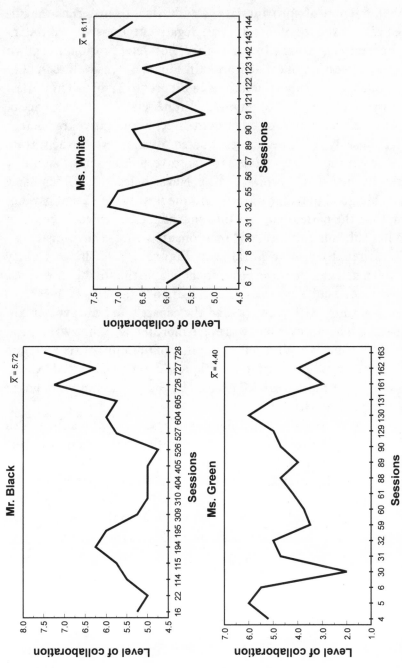

Figure 6–3. Changes in Luborsky Type II therapeutic alliance across sessions.

Type I alliance that Ms. Green maintained could be viewed as an epiphenomenon of splitting (i.e., an idealized transference maintained at the expense of directing all negative feelings toward the inpatient treatment team). In this regard, her deterioration, as shown by our own measure of collaboration in Figure 6–1, as well as in both Type I and Type II Luborsky ratings in Figures 6–2 and 6–3 in the last few sessions of the psychotherapy, might be related to the absence of other treaters toward whom she could direct her negative transferential feelings. By the time she terminated psychotherapy, she was no longer in an inpatient setting and had divested herself of ancillary treaters in the partial hospital setting. Nevertheless, Ms. Green had a reasonably good outcome overall, and the positive effects of psychotherapy on the patient suggest that she may have derived some gain from her split-off and idealized relationship with the therapist.

Another difference notable in Figure 6–3 is the difficulty Ms. Green had in sustaining positive changes in the alliance measures. This same difficulty is reflected in Figure 6–1 in our own measures of collaboration. Although she had the capacity to improve her collaboration, the improvement was much more tenuous than was typical of Mr. Black and Ms. White. This fragility of the ability to collaborate may require more supportive techniques, as reflected in the expressive-supportive measures used to rate Ms. Green's therapy as opposed to the other two cases.

Ms. Green's difficulty in collaborating with her therapist is also evident on examining changes in collaboration *within* sessions. Table 6–4 suggests that in a typical session, Mr. Black or Ms. White increased their collaboration with the therapist approximately one-half of a scale point.

On the other hand, Ms. Green tended to show little or no change in collaboration. The same struggles to work with the therapist toward

Table 6–4. Mean level of change in collaboration within sessions (first to last third)

Mr. Black	Ms. Green	Ms. White
.50	.08	.47

mutually embraced goals can be noted by comparing the three patients in terms of the percentage of sessions that were characterized by changes in collaboration (see Table 6–5).

In the psychotherapeutic processes of Mr. Black and Ms. White, more than 70% of their sessions that were rated showed increases in collaboration. By contrast, Ms. Green's collaboration with her therapist increased in only a third of the sessions rated. In 44% of her sessions, no change was noted, and in 22% of Ms. Green's sessions, the collaboration deteriorated, a development that was uncommon with Ms. White and unheard of with Mr. Black.

Process Analysis

Having described the three psychotherapies on a more global level, we now turn to a detailed analysis of the process of each case. As the ratings reflect, the psychotherapy of Mr. Black was by far the most expressive of the three. From early in the treatment, there was a consistent focus on the transference and a liberal use of transference interpretations. These interventions appeared to be instrumental in producing increased collaboration during the first half of the psychotherapy. Mr. Black's therapist also used confrontations involving the transference early in the therapy, and these were also viewed as significant factors in increasing the patient's collaboration. Contrary to the impressions of Gunderson's group (Frank 1992; Gunderson et al. 1989), these early transference-focused interventions did not result in the patient's dropping out of therapy or even in significant deterioration in the collaboration. Unlike some borderline patients,

Table 6–5.   Percentage of sessions with beginning-to-end changes in collaboration

	Mr. Black	Ms. Green	Ms. White
Increases	71	33	78
No change	29	44	11
Decreases	0	22	11

Mr. Black did not respond to transference-based interventions as though they were attacks that required heightened defensiveness, retaliation, or flight.

The patient's powerful unconscious conviction that he was deserving of punishment, subjugation, and humiliation was associated with masochistic sexual fantasies. Although at a conscious level he was using the therapist's insight to promote deepened understanding of himself, unconsciously he may have experienced interventions and confrontations as a sadomasochistic enactment with the therapist from which he derived a masochistic form of transference gratification. In this regard, the diminution of transference-based interventions and confrontations in the latter part of the therapy can be understood as reflecting the working through of the sadomasochistic conflicts, the internalization of the therapist's activity, and the modification of Mr. Black's superego.

It is also of note that even though nontransference interventions tended to increase collaboration in the latter half of the therapy and transference interventions decreased in number and frequency, the supportive and expressive scores remained consistent. Although psychoanalytic psychotherapists tend to associate expressive treatments with transference-focused treatment, interpretations targeted at extratransference phenomena can also form the basis of expressive work.

The vast majority of the shifts in collaboration noted within sessions (89%) occurred in an upward direction in Mr. Black's psychotherapy, and 63% of these could be linked to focus on the transference relationship. However, all four of the downward shifts in collaboration were *also* linked to transference interventions. Those that produced deteriorations in the collaborative relationship with the therapist were often assessed by the raters as too long, too direct, lacking in empathy, and overly confrontational. The log linear analysis (see Appendix C) also documented a significant relationship between transference-focused interventions and downward shifts. One striking conclusion from our analysis of the process was that transference-focused interventions have a consistently greater impact than nontransference interventions. *Both* kinds of shifts in collaboration —upward and downward—are more likely to occur with transference-based comments. Stated simply, transference interventions are high-risk, high-gain comments.

In the case of Ms. Green, her well-honed verbal skills, her superficial social adaptation, and a certain pseudosophistication about psychological matters led both the therapist and the independent judges to overestimate her ability to use an expressive process. The "honeymoon phase" of the psychotherapy rapidly gave way to a stance of "having one foot out the door," requiring a good deal of therapist activity to keep Ms. Green engaged in the process. The therapist revised his initial ambitions for an expressive approach and was able to shift to supportive techniques that were more suited to the patient. This psychotherapy was the only one of the three rated more supportive than expressive.

In stark contrast to Mr. Black's psychotherapy, only 29% of the upward shifts in Ms. Green's collaboration could be related to transference-focused interventions. By and large, interpretations of negative transference led to avoidance and externalization. In the last third of the psychotherapy, the therapist had clearly learned to adapt to the patient's needs by eliminating almost all interpretive and transference-focused interventions.

Examination of those instances in which transference interventions did improve the alliance revealed that they were almost always preceded by multiple supportive interventions. This approach is very much in keeping with Pine's (1984) advice that with seriously disturbed patients, one may need to provide a holding environment while offering an interpretation. This notion of interpretation within the context of support emphasizes that the supportive-expressive issue is not an either-or proposition, as we note in Chapter 1 (this volume). Indeed, the provision of support creates an ambience in which the patient can listen to and reflect on observations that may be otherwise experienced as narcissistically injurious.

A recurrent struggle in the therapy of Ms. Green was to get her to reflect on her own contribution to difficulties whose origins she had externalized and on particular acting-out behaviors. Therapists often approach such material with the conviction that therapy is based on such an examination, and they can become highly frustrated, as Ms. Green's therapist did, when the patient will not collaborate in the introspective process. Gunderson (1992) candidly described his own reaction to a patient who would not join him in examining her behavior:

As an analytic therapist I felt that such examining was what I was being paid for, what I was good at, and what I liked to do. It was easy to lose sight of the fact that behaviorally she was generally doing much better and to infer that she was under a lot of added stress from recently resuming school. Rather than actively supporting her I was getting preoccupied with the fact that she would not/could not look at herself with me. (p. 303)

In some cases the patient's recalcitrance toward the therapist's efforts to make the patient think psychologically about behavior and experience may result in an escalating and counterproductive string of transference interpretations. In one study that linked transference interpretation to the therapeutic alliance in outcome, Piper et al. (1991) found that in a subgroup of patients, an increased frequency of transference interpretations was associated with poor therapeutic alliance and negative outcome. Although these investigators were not studying borderline patients, their findings about the lack of success in resolving impasses with the use of transference interpretation may be applicable to psychotherapy of borderline patients. They noted that the patient's negative transference elicits a high proportion of transference interpretations, leading to the patient's further resistance until the psychotherapy falls into alternating cycles of silence and transference interpretation.

An examination of the types of supportive interventions that were useful in the therapy of Ms. Green suggest that first and foremost, the therapist's high level of verbal activity was experienced by the patient as holding and containment. Affirmation and validation of her internal experience also seemed to increase her ability to collaborate. In the third audiotaped vignette described in Chapter 4 (this volume), the therapist did not challenge Ms. Green's tendency to externalize responsibility for that which was negative, and he noted that "it certainly is to your credit that you're managing to face all this tension now." The combination of his tolerance of her externalization and his affirmation of her struggle allowed her to talk more openly about how she valued his help and the therapy in general. Paradoxically, his supportive focus on extratransference issues also seemed to improve the patient's capacity to speak more openly about the relationship with the therapist.

Ms. Green was prone to action rather than reflectiveness. Help was most concretely conceptualized as coming in the form of a pill. Her action proneness within the psychotherapy was most frequently manifested in her "one-foot-out-the-door" stance (i.e., her wish to take flight from the therapy). This stance evoked a countertransference pressure in Ms. Green's therapist to act. He felt he was constantly pursuing her and trying to focus and clarify her scattered thoughts and her half-formed plans of action. This heightened verbal activity and pursuit of her in response to her wish to escape may well have provided a partial transference gratification for Ms. Green. She felt that her therapist was involved and engaged and was not abandoning her even when she was most negative about the treatment. This level of activity created countertransference anxiety in Ms. Green's therapist because he felt he was not being sufficiently expressive, particularly in light of the case being tape recorded. The bias of most psychotherapists toward expressive work—and the fantasy of what *other* therapists might think about shifting to supportive technique—cannot be underestimated as a significant influence on the therapist's conduct of psychotherapy with borderline patients. Therapists clearly need permission to shift from an expressive to a supportive approach when warranted without feeling guilty about it. The fact remains that most borderline patients require and receive a predominantly supportive psychotherapy (Rockland 1992). As noted earlier, when Ms. Green's partial hospital team disappeared from the picture, her splitting defense was more difficult to maintain, and the therapist became less idealized. Her alliance deteriorated near the end of therapy as she continued to insist on quitting in opposition to her therapist's assertion that she needed to continue. She did follow through with her plans to leave and ultimately had a reasonably good outcome. At follow-up she was assessed to be less psychologically minded and insightful than before, but her functioning was clearly improved.

One way to understand the patient's improvement is related to Wallerstein's (1986) observation from his study of the Menninger Foundation Psychotherapy Research Project (PRP) outcomes. One group that ultimately did well were characterized by an "antitransference cure," in which they defied their therapists by getting better. In the McLean study of therapeutic alliance with borderline patients (Frank 1992), one subgroup developed a "negative-oppositional" alliance in which they were highly engaged with their therapists through a process of struggling about every aspect of the treatment. More than half stayed in psychotherapy for 9 months or more, and they eventually were able to use treatment to their advantage. The patients became convinced that the therapists could survive their rage and defiance. Similar mechanisms may have been at work in the outcome of Ms. Green.

Ms. White's therapy process was regarded as intermediate between Mr. Black's and Ms. Green's in terms of the expressive-supportive dimension. Like Ms. Green, Ms. White developed a split transference in which the therapist was the idealized pole. The patient's rage at the therapist was displaced from the transference onto Ms. White's husband. Also like Ms. Green, she apparently derived some benefit from the idealized view of the therapist. Her self-experience and self-esteem seemed to be enhanced by identifying with the idealized image of the therapist.

One of the major differences between Ms. White and Ms. Green is that Ms. White was able to use a much more expressive approach than Ms. Green. Of the upward shifts in collaboration that could be linked to therapist interventions, 81% resulted from a transference focus by the therapist. However, an examination of pivotal interventions that increased collaboration suggested that most of them took place in the context of a long series of interventions that had a cumulative effect. The therapist's attunement to the patient's emotional state seemed to create a therapeutic climate that fostered expressive work. Pine's (1984) notion of interpreting within the context of support appeared to be just as relevant to Ms. White as it was to Ms. Green.

A corollary of this finding is that we should avoid artificially isolating transference interpretations but rather should consider them as part of a series of interventions. Indeed, in a process study of two anxious and depressed women in brief dynamic therapy, Messer et al. (1992) found that researchers should not expect individual interventions to produce patient response in a highly predictable manner. Rather, they found that the cumulative effect of a number of individual interventions over time was more predictable.

Transference-related interventions were also linked to 80% of those downward shifts in collaboration that could actually be linked to any comment by the therapist. These interventions that caused worsening in the patient's collaborative ability tended to grow out of the therapist's lack of attunement to the patient's emotional state or a miscalculation regarding the amount of intense affect that the patient could tolerate. Once again, the role of transference interventions as "high-risk, high-gain" propositions was confirmed.

One factor that may partly determine the success of the transference interpretation is the suitability of the intervention for the particular patient. Silberschatz et al. (1986) studied the process of three brief psychodynamic therapies with nonborderline patients and found that in each case suitability of the interpretation correlated significantly with patient expectation. Specifically, they looked at suitability in the context of whether the interpretation was consistent with the patient's unconscious plan with which he or she approached psychotherapy, as described by Weiss (1993). In this formulation, developed by Weiss and Sampson at the Mt. Zion Psychotherapy Research Project, an interpretation may be accurate, but it may not be experienced as helpful unless it gives the patient something that he or she unconsciously wants to receive as part of his or her individual plan. For example, the patient may approach the therapy with an unconscious goal of disconfirming that male authority figures are critical. If the therapist interprets this dynamic in the transference, the patient will feel understood. In this regard, the important distinction is not between transference and nontransference interpretation, but between proplan and antiplan interpretations (Weiss 1993).

Similar findings emerge from a different model, the core conflictual relationship theme method of Luborsky and Crits-Christoph (1990). In a study of 33 patients in psychodynamic treatments of moderate length (Crits-Christoph et al. 1993), the researchers found that accuracy of interpretation on a key dimension of this method (the patient's wish or intention toward others and the desired response of others) strongly predicted positive changes in the therapeutic alliance. Although the members of the interventions subgroup in our study rated the suitability of each interpretation, the ratings did not vary sufficiently to draw any conclusions about the relationship between suitability and collaboration.

Sigal (1993) suggested that gender may also influence the response to transference interpretations. When Piper et al. (1993) reanalyzed their study in response to a letter by Sigal, their data suggested that males may have a relatively positive reaction to high levels of transference interpretations whereas females have a negative reaction. Further research needs to be done to determine whether this is a consistent finding. Although our own data correlate with the observations of Piper et al., the small number of patients in our sample precludes any definitive conclusions.

Early in the second half of Ms. White's psychotherapy process, the Luborsky Type I measure of the therapeutic alliance appeared to worsen (see Figure 6–2), suggesting that the patient's idealized transference toward the therapist faltered. In the midst of an apparent crisis, the therapist became more supportive and uncharacteristically gave a great deal of advice and praise. Nevertheless, the degree of expressiveness did not decline during this crisis, and expressive interventions such as interpretation and confrontation continued. Greater support was necessary to help bolster the patient's affect tolerance so that the expressive interventions could be heard and understood. The therapist also postponed interpretation of negative transference until the elaboration of transference metaphors had been fostered through supportive interventions.

A striking similarity between Ms. White and Ms. Green reveals itself in their response to their therapist's efforts to make them more reflective and internally oriented when they were experiencing strong affect toward a third party and were therefore *externally* oriented. Both patients tenaciously resisted efforts to help them look inward and maintained their insistence that their problems were outside them. In both processes, when the therapist could in some way affirm their internal experience of the other person, the patients' collaboration ultimately improved.

Like Ms. Green, Ms. White spent much of the therapy wanting to reduce the frequency of the sessions and/or terminate. In fact, she preferred sealing over rather than expanding insight. The independent judges assessed her as somewhat less psychologically minded and insightful after the therapy than before (like Ms. Green), and she was seen as reaching premature closure on a number of her basic conflicts. Nevertheless, her gains from identifying with the therapist and feeling understood and affirmed appeared to pay off in substantial improvements after therapy had terminated.

Patient Characteristics and the Expressive-Supportive Dimension

To make our findings in this intensive study of three cases useful to psychotherapists treating other borderline patients, it is essential for us to identify patient characteristics that can be linked to suitability for varying degrees of expressive and supportive technique. An examination of the characteristics of Mr. Black, Ms. Green, and Ms. White suggests that each represents a different subtype of borderline patient. Mr. Black has many of the characteristics described by Grinker et al. (1968) as Type IV or "neurotic border." His depressive tendencies were largely anaclitic in nature, his anxiety had many elements in common with neurotic anxiety, and he had narcissistic and masochistic features as well. Ms. Green fits well within Grinker's Type II, the "core borderline syndrome." She showed vacillating involvement with others, pervasive anger and negative affect, and a confused self-identity. Finally, Ms. White resembled Grinker's Type III, the "as-if group," in that her uncertainty about her identity led her to develop a false self so that her relationships lacked spontaneity and genuineness. Her behavior and functioning were in general more adaptive than many borderline patients as well. In this regard, we should emphasize that she managed to avoid hospitalization, even in the midst of a crisis, in contrast to Mr. Black and Ms. Green, who spent large amounts of their psychotherapy on inpatient units. She also was able to hold a good job and tolerate the intimacy of marriage.

In considering the diagnoses of our three patients, we were puzzled that they met DSM-III-R (American Psychiatric Association 1987) criteria for borderline personality disorder but not those of the Diagnostic Interview for Borderline Patients (DIB) (Gunderson et al. 1981). In a study of the test-retest reliability of the instrument, Cornell et al. (1983) found that extensive training was necessary to establish reliability. Our raters did not receive rigorous training, and that factor may account for the low DIB scores. Also, rating from videotapes reduces the affective intensity one feels with borderline patients in the consulting room and may affect ratings as well.

Although Grinker et al.'s (1968) categories are useful, more detailed assessments of developmental factors, ego factors, and relationship factors are necessary to characterize similarities and differences among our patients more specifically.

Developmental Factors

In the case of Mr. Black, the key developmental factors in which we were interested were largely absent. Although he did not suffer from any extraordinary traumas, he was subjected to the developmental strain of a relatively absent father and a mother who demeaned males as uncontrollable beasts. On the other hand, no neurological dysfunction was present. By contrast, developmental factors appeared to be of considerable importance in the etiology and pathogenesis of Ms. Green's difficulties. A strong case could be made for a constitutional hyperirritability of her central nervous system, an etiological factor observed by Stone (1993) in significant numbers of borderline patients. Neuropsychological testing documented numerous erratic cognitive deficits, including spatial orientation problems, visual-spatial and semantic memory problems, difficulties with left-right discrimination, fine-motor coordination problems, and difficulty shifting cognitive sets.

When Ms. Green was a baby, her parents' extraordinary efforts could not contain her hyperactivity. They ultimately resorted to practices that were undoubtedly highly traumatic to her, such as wedging her door shut and allowing her to scream frantically until she fell asleep. She likely felt abandoned in a state of high arousal. This bit of historical data underscores an important premise in understanding the etiology of borderline personality disorder—constitutional and traumatic factors may well coexist and work synergistically to produce the end result of borderline personality disorder. Too often the search for historical influences leads to an unproductive either-or philosophy that the patient is either the victim of trauma or temperamentally difficult.

Ms. White was not neurologically compromised in any way but had some early trauma. She felt obligated to protect her mother from her father's violence, and her parentified childhood role led to an as-if quality in her assumption of the pseudo-self-sufficient caretaker persona. Table 6–6 summarizes the developmental characteristics of the three patients.

Table 6–6. Developmental factors

	Early trauma	Neurological dysfunction
Mr. Black	None	None
Ms. Green	Parental abandonment at bedtime	Erratic cognitive deficits
Ms. White	Parentified child who protected mother from father's violence	None

Patients with neurologically based cognitive dysfunction may have difficulty with the abstract thinking necessary to work expressively. Interpretations may thus produce feelings of shame and humiliation that they cannot grasp the therapist's meaning. Supportive technique is clearly much more effective, as shown in the therapy of Ms. Green. Similarly, a history of childhood trauma may require a specific type of supportive technique. Patients who have experienced trauma are likely to persist in viewing others as aggressive and persecutory. This externalization of the source of aggression needs to be empathized with and validated for the patient to feel held. If the patient's aggression is prematurely dealt with as primary and internal, the patient will feel misunderstood and unable to collaborate with the therapist. Our observations are in keeping with the shift in approach to borderline patients that has resulted from the recognition of the significant role that trauma plays in the etiology of borderline personality disorder (Gunderson and Sabo 1993). Within this new framework, the patient's aggression is understood as a reasonable reaction to parents who fail to deal with a child's emotional needs or who cruelly use the child for their own needs. Another implication is that hateful or rage-filled transferences must be contained and tolerated rather than prematurely interpreted as growing out of the patient's own difficulties (Epstein 1979; Gabbard 1991).

Ego Factors

Motivation for change. The three patients differ considerably in their motivation to use psychotherapy as a means for constructive change. Mr. Black was highly motivated to find relief for his suffering through a better understanding of himself. Ms. Green, on the other hand, had limited motivation. She tended to view insight as unimportant. Her primary wish was to get immediate gratification in the form of a pill or a relationship. In the case of Ms. White, her suicidal depressive crisis and bulimia made her motivated to seek treatment, but she had greater difficulty sustaining that motivation in times of crisis or when the relationship with the therapist felt uncomfortably close.

Capacity to work in an analytic space.   Mr. Black's capacity to generate personal meanings in the transference and experience the therapist "as if" he were someone else while reflecting on the process was well developed so that psychotic transference distortions were rare or absent. In the case of Ms. Green, there was a collapse of analytic space for the most part so that she was unable to reflect on her transference experiences as they were occurring. Ms. White was once again in between Mr. Black and Ms. Green, in the sense that her capacity to enter into an analytic space with her therapist was more variable and limited than Mr. Black but greater than Ms. Green.

Impulse control and affect tolerance.   The three patients line up in the same way regarding impulse control and affect tolerance. Mr. Black, although prone to suicidal ideation, was able to delay impulse discharge and modulate affective states. Ms. Green was quite impaired in her ability to regulate affect and to control impulses. Ms. White was somewhere in between the two; she could tolerate dysphoric states, but intense rage and envy were hard for her to manage, and her bulimia reflected some difficulties with impulse control.

Proneness to externalization.   Most patients with borderline personality disorder will at times externalize their difficulties and blame others. Although Mr. Black occasionally viewed the world in this way, for the most part he had the capacity to perceive his difficulties as originating within him. In his masochistic orientation, he tended to blame himself even when sadistically mistreated by others. By contrast, Ms. Green consistently saw her difficulties arising as a result of the mistreatment by others, most notably in her attitude about the inpatient treatment team. Ms. White presented a mixed picture; she blamed her husband a great deal for her suffering, but she also manifested self-criticism and self-blame, particularly around her failures to save her siblings.

Psychological-mindedness. Mr. Black was clearly the most psychologically sophisticated in his ability to think abstractly and symbolically about his behavior and experience. Although Ms. Green initially presented a sophisticated facade, her capacity for reflection was severely limited, perhaps in part related to her cognitive dysfunction. Ms. White initially demonstrated psychological-mindedness to a fairly impressive degree, but as she fled the therapy, she became increasingly concrete. The ego factors characteristic of the three different patients are summarized in Table 6–7.

A comparison of the ego factors characteristic of Mr. Black, Ms. Green, and Ms. White clearly shows a consistent pattern. On all five measures, Mr. Black rated the highest, Ms. Green the lowest, and Ms. White between the two. These five factors, then, compellingly reflect the capacity of the three patients to use expressive versus supportive interventions. Mr. Black's therapy was the most expressive, Ms. Green's was the most supportive, and Ms. White required a mixture of expressive and supportive techniques. These ego factors were apparent to the independent judges, even without the extensive data of the psychotherapy sessions, suggesting that such an assessment can be made with some degree of accuracy as part of an initial evaluation.

Relationship Factors

Narcissistic vulnerability. Mr. Black was able to tolerate observations by the therapist without feeling devastated. Possibly because of his masochistic tendencies, interpretations that may have been experienced critically were also gratifying to him. Ms. Green's fragile self-esteem made her highly vulnerable to any comment by the therapist that could be experienced as critical in any way. She had a long-standing pattern of falling short of expectations (perhaps because of her cognitive limitations) and was therefore prone to shame and humiliation. Ms. White was also narcissistically vulnerable and shame-prone. Transference wishes involving dependency and sexual feelings

Table 6–7. Ego factors

	Motivation	Capacity for analytic space	Impulse control/ affect tolerance	Proneness to externalization	Psychological-mindedness
Mr. Black	High	Good	Reasonably good, but suicidal	Limited	Exceptional
Ms. Green	Low	Poor	Poor	Extreme	Limited
Ms. White	Variable	Limited and variable	Variable	Mixed picture	Variable

evoked intense embarrassment, and speaking openly about her needs for affirmation from the therapist were deeply troubling.

Mirroring and idealizing transferences. All three patients showed some idealization in the transference. Mr. Black was defensive against his unacceptable competitiveness and aggression. Ms. Green formed a split-off, idealized transference that coexisted with her negative transference to the inpatient staff. Later in the treatment, a mirroring transference, in which she longed for admiration and acceptance from her therapist to bolster her self-esteem, became more prominent. Ms. Green clearly needed the therapist's empathic attunement to maintain a sense of self-cohesion, as described by Kohut (1971). In Ms. White's search for an affirming parent who would serve her developmental needs, she longed for mirroring from her therapist but also idealized him at times.

Distancing and counterdependency. Although Mr. Black began the treatment by using obsessional defenses to maintain distance, he eventually overcame his fears of closeness and made his powerful wishes for emotional intimacy apparent to the therapist. Ms. Green's stance of wanting to flee treatment reflected extreme counterdependency. Ms. White was also markedly counterdependent, wearing self-sufficiency as a badge throughout her life.

Clinging and symbiotic needs. Mr. Black longed for parental approval and succor but was too conflicted about his dependent longings to manifest clinging or symbiotic yearnings. Ms. Green maintained an overtly counterdependent stance but acted in ways that made others pursue her in a way she perceived as clinging. This projective disavowal allowed her to reassure herself that others were dependent on her while she was independent. Ms. White was so deeply ashamed of any dependency wishes that clinging or symbiotic needs did not surface.

Sadistic and erotized transferences. Mr. Black's perception of the therapist as his partner in a sadomasochistic enactment was a major part of the therapeutic work. Neither sadistic nor erotized transferences entered into the psychotherapy relationship with Ms. Green, but she certainly perceived other treaters as sadistic. Ms. White also did not experience any overt sadistic or erotized elements in her transference relationship to the therapist. From time to time, however, there were hints that sexual feelings were being suppressed.

Capacity for concern. Both Mr. Black and Ms. White manifested a good deal of concern about others. Both were aware of their capacity to harm others, and Ms. White in particular chastised herself for her personal failings that had caused harm to others. A major theme of her life was making reparation to those she had harmed. Ms. Green was more overtly angry and less concerned about her capacity to harm others. However, she did feel extremely guilty about what she had put her parents through and feared hurting them further. Table 6–8 summarizes the similarities in relationship factors among the three patients.

The relationship factors show much less variability than the ego factors. The extreme narcissistic vulnerability present in both Ms. Green and Ms. White was clearly instrumental in their needing more supportive techniques than Mr. Black, whose self-esteem was somewhat more durable. On the closeness and distance dimensions, the patients were more alike than different. However, the flexibility hypothesis stated in Chapter 1 (this volume) was largely confirmed in the study of these three cases. Of all the patients, Mr. Black could move most flexibly within the closeness-distance spectrum, particularly as the therapy proceeded. In keeping with our hypothesis, he was also the one most able to use expressive work. Ms. Green, on the other hand, was incapable of closeness with the therapist and steadfastly maintained a distant, counterdependent stance and required the most supportive technique of the three cases. Finally, Ms. White allowed herself only moments of closeness, but for the most part maintained a counterdependent stance as well. She was able to use expressive interventions to some degree, but only with considerable accompanying support.

Mechanisms of Change

In considering what factors are mutative in the psychotherapy of borderline patients, the expressive versus supportive controversy often

Table 6–8. Relationship factors

	Narcissistic vulnerability	Mirroring/ idealizing transference	Distancing and counterdependency	Clinging/ symbiotic needs	Sadistic/ erotized transference	Capacity for concern
Mr. Black	Limited	Defensive idealization	Obsessional defenses to avoid closeness	Not apparent	Sadistic	Present
Ms. Green	Extreme	Idealization early, mirroring late	Extreme counter-dependency	Projective disavowal	None	Present
Ms. White	Extreme	Idealizing and mirroring	Extreme counterdependency	Not apparent	None	Limited

gets cast in terms of insight versus relationship. Does interpretation of unconscious conflict produce structural change (the conflict model), or is internalization of a new relationship with the therapist (the deficit model) responsible for change? These two agents of psychotherapeutic change often get polarized in the same manner as the expressive versus supportive dimensions. The emphasis may be more in one direction than the other with any given patient, but in most cases some combination of the two are at work. A new interpersonal relationship may in and of itself produce insight (Cooper 1992), and the understanding of a relationship may be necessary to maintain it (Pulver 1992).

According to research (Blatt 1990, 1992; Blatt and Behrens 1987), one subtype of patients may be more responsive to interpretive interventions and insight, whereas another subtype may gain greater therapeutic value from the quality of the therapeutic relationship. These two subtypes have been described, respectively, as *introjective* and *anaclitic*. Patients with anaclitic psychopathology are more concerned with issues of relatedness than self-development and use avoidant defenses such as denial, disavowal, withdrawal, repression, and displacement. Patients with introjective psychopathology, on the other hand, are more ideational and are primarily preoccupied with establishing and maintaining a viable self-concept than with establishing intimacy in the interpersonal realm. Their principal defenses are intellectualization, reaction formation, rationalization, doing and undoing, and projection. Although both anaclitic and introjective patients are found in the borderline continuum, the overideational borderline patients, such as Mr. Black, appear to be more responsive to insight and interpretation, whereas anaclitic patients, such as Ms. Green, are more responsive to the interpersonal dimensions of the psychotherapeutic process. This differential response, however, is relative rather than absolute, and Blatt (1992) acknowledged that most patients undoubtedly benefit from both aspects of the therapeutic interaction.

In the psychotherapy of Ms. Green, insight seemed to be far less important than the relationship with her psychotherapist, but some expressive comments could be productive as long as an environment of support had been created. Similarly, Ms. White also required her therapist's empathic attunement as a preexisting context for her to receive and reflect on interpretive interventions. Less preparatory support was needed for Mr. Black to benefit from interpretations. Mr. Black attributed the punitive quality of his "savage superego" to the therapist and was therefore inhibited about revealing aggressive and sexual concerns in the sessions. He seemed to fear that opening up about such concerns would lead to the therapist's retaliation and ridicule. Transference interpretations were helpful because they clarified the patient's fears in the here and now, giving permission for the patient to explore his anxiety-laden material. These interpretations were mutative in the sense that they helped Mr. Black realize that his fear derived from internal and irrational sources rather than from real and external threats. He could then see the therapist as a helping person with whom he could safely collaborate, resulting in an internalization of a more benign parental figure. That introjection process, in turn, made a significant alteration in Mr. Black's superego, illustrating the convergence of both interpretive and relationship factors.

Our intensive study of these three cases lead us to much the same conclusion reached by Waldinger and Gunderson (1987) in their study of five successfully treated patients with borderline personality disorder. They found that no one specific theory or technique holds the answer for all borderline patients. Early transference work is clearly effective with some but not with others. Validation of internal states may be particularly useful with borderline patients who are trauma victims but not particularly helpful with those who are not.

There is growing recognition that supportive techniques may be instrumental to the change process with many borderline patients (Gunderson and Sabo 1993; Rockland 1992). Two of the psychotherapies in our project, those of Ms. Green and Ms. White, began with an expressive orientation, only to shift in a more supportive direction as the patients required it. In both Horwitz's (1974) and Wallerstein's (1986) examinations of the PRP cases, they found a similar trend in the treatment of disturbed patients who would now be diagnosed as borderline in many cases. They identified several mechanisms of change in such patients. A transference cure effected through an unanalyzed positive dependent transference seemed to be at work in some. In keeping with Horwitz's earlier conclusions, our findings suggest that even if that unanalyzed positive dependent transference is one pole of a split, there still may be therapeutic gains deriving from it. As noted earlier, Wallerstein also identified the antitransference cure, which involved changing by defying the therapist. The mechanism may, in part, account for some of Ms. Green's improvements.

Both Horwitz (1974) and Wallerstein (1986) concluded that a variant of the corrective emotional experience in which the patient's transference behavior is met by the therapist with nonjudgmental, nonretaliatory responses, the reverse of what was expected, may also be an important factor. Still other patients responded to friendly advice and educational interventions.

Rockland (1992), who maintained that the majority of borderline patients require predominantly supportive approaches, described mechanisms of change that are similar to Wallerstein's (1986) categories. In addition, he has noted that the systematic strengthening of the patient's ego functions may produce lasting change. Rockland observed that some patients become less paranoid because of positive interactions with a therapist only to then find that other people also begin to respond in more supportive and trusting ways. These extratransference interactions allow the patient to become even less paranoid, creating a positive feedback loop between the transference and relationships outside the transference.

In our examination of the transcripts, we also observed another mechanism of change that occurs over and over again in the psychotherapy of borderline patients. We repeatedly noted a *repair process,* involving active work by therapist and patient to repair a breakdown or rupture of the therapeutic alliance. The repair of these ruptures, whether done through interpretation or some other combination of interventions, seemed to have a cumulative effect resulting in positive outcome. Our observations confirm the view that psychotherapy is a process that proceeds in a series of separations followed by attachments, what Blatt and Behrens (1987) referred to as "experienced incompatibilities" and "gratifying involvements." These ruptures in the alliance followed by their repair gradually build up a new view of the self in relation to others and more mature levels of psychological structures. This new view, then, becomes internalized and eventually may be considered to reflect structural change.

We were somewhat surprised to observe that in all three cases the patients' collaboration did not show substantive improvement from the beginning to the end of the psychotherapy. The McLean study (Frank 1992) also met with some difficulty in demonstrating a unique contribution of the therapeutic alliance to outcome. For purposes of convenience and the possibility of arriving at reasonable interrater consensus, we narrowed the complex concept of the therapeutic alliance to a relatively specific marker—collaboration. As Allen et al. (1988) and Frank (1992) noted, in multiple-treater situations, such as hospital or day hospital settings, there may be multiple alliances, each with multiple dimensions independent of one another. By narrowing our focus to the study of collaboration, we may be measuring a partial or incomplete therapeutic alliance. By specifically relating collaboration to the bringing in of significant new information and making use of the therapist's comments, we narrowed the definition of collaboration further. However, our observation of the rupture-repair process in tracking the patient's collaboration convinces us of the usefulness of the alliance concept.

There is no question that using written transcripts of audiotaped sessions excludes certain data from the raters that are available to a psychotherapist. For example, the affective tone conveyed by the patient's voice and the nonverbal communication telegraphed by body movements are not available to the rater. However, as Gill (1982) argued, verbatim transcripts are far superior for examination of microscopic process details than summaries recalled from memory by the therapist. Although videotapes would provide more information, they are certainly much more intrusive than a tape recorder sitting on a table.

Despite the limitations of our measure of collaboration in capturing the complexities of the therapeutic alliance, we nevertheless feel that the alliance is a useful construct for the psychotherapist working with borderline patients. We strongly disagree with Adler's (1992) view that the alliance is a myth. He believes that the selfobject bond is too tenuous and easily decimated by narcissistic rage and fragmentation to be useful. He further cautions that the therapist's wish to have the patient collaborate may be perceived by the patient as a demand that cannot be fulfilled and therefore an empathic failure of the therapist. By contrast, clinical observation of our cases revealed that the repair of the moment-to-moment disruptions in the alliance often was a key factor in maintaining the viability of the psychotherapy. The internalization of this repair process involves an identification with the therapist that is also central to change with borderline patients. This observation supports Horwitz's (1974) suggestion that internalization of the therapeutic alliance may be an important mechanism of change in supportive psychotherapy of borderline patients.

Many of the ruptures in the alliance stem directly from transference-countertransference enactments. Through projective identification, borderline patients tend to evoke responses in therapists that correspond to internal self and object representations within the patient. The retrospective examination of these countertransference responses with the patient provides a great deal of diagnostic data about the patient's internal world (Gabbard and Wilkinson 1994). Thus, the systematic analysis and management of one's countertransference responses become crucial to the repair and maintenance of the therapeutic alliance.

Conclusions

The primary value of all psychotherapy research is to use the data to derive conclusions that can be generalized to other patients and other psychotherapy processes. A major concern, of course, is the degree of generalizability with the intensive case study design. Will *all* borderline patients with characteristics of Ms. Green, for example, respond as she did to transference interpretations? We cannot make definitive predictions that apply to all patients. Only randomized controlled trials of manualized therapies for different subgroups of borderline patients would answer such questions, and even this method may fall short insofar as all subgroups are characterized by high degrees of interindividual variability. However, intensive study of individual cases reveals information about the microscopic details of process that controlled studies with large samples fail to address. Indeed, the two methodologies complement one another.

Recognizing the limitations of our method, we nevertheless offer a series of conclusions that may be useful to clinicians involved in the treatment of borderline patients. These conclusions may also serve as hypotheses that could be tested in future research with larger samples.

Borderline patients are not a monolithic group.   We share the view of Meissner (1984, 1988) and Grinker et al. (1968) that a spectrum of borderline conditions exist. The different subtypes along the spectrum require different psychotherapeutic strategies. Moreover, there is now a broad consensus that multiple etiological and pathogenetic factors contribute to the final common pathway of borderline personality disorder (Gabbard 1994; Paris and Zweig-Frank 1992; Zanarini et al. 1989). These diverse factors (such as trauma, loss, and constitutional dispositions) must be taken into account in treatment planning.

No single psychotherapeutic approach is suited for all borderline patients. This point, of course, follows directly from our first conclusion. Most of the therapeutic approaches described in the literature are useful for *some* patients *some* of the time. A careful assessment of the developmental factors, ego factors, relationship factors, and the patient's ability to shift flexibly between closeness and distance is of considerable value in designing a particular therapeutic strategy for a particular patient.

Shifting flexibly from expressive to supportive techniques is essential in the psychotherapy of borderline patients. In agreement with Horwitz's (1974) and Wallerstein's (1986) findings, our analysis of the data suggests that clinicians are often overly ambitious in their wish to apply expressive techniques to borderline patients. To some extent, this tendency grows out of a bias toward expressive psychotherapy deriving from the psychoanalytic tradition. Therapists of borderline patients must feel an inner sense of freedom or permission to shift from expressive to supportive approaches, or to bolster expressive interventions with supportive ones, according to the moment-to-moment requirements of the patient. In fact, in L. Horwitz's ("Therapist Personality and Level of Competence," unpublished manuscript, May 1971) comparison of high- and low-skill therapists in the PRP, flexibility in adjusting the therapy to the patient's responses was a major differentiating factor.

Expressive and supportive interventions should not be juxtaposed as polarized opposites—they often work synergistically. Supportive comments create a therapeutic climate in which the patient can tolerate interpretations and reflect on their personal meanings. As noted by Pine (1984) and Gunderson (1992), interpretation that takes place in a supportive ambience makes possible an expansion of the range of patients who can benefit from insight.

Transference interpretations should be regarded as high-risk, high-gain interventions. Disagreements in the literature regarding the value of transference interpretations with borderline patients may reflect the tendency for these comments to have greater impact—both positive and negative—than other interventions made with borderline patients. Therapists should carefully weigh the state of the therapeutic alliance before attempting transference interpretations. As Meissner (1988) pointed out, the intactness of the therapeutic alliance is the prerequisite for interpretive work.

Partial transference gratifications are inevitable and often therapeutic in the psychotherapy of borderline patients.   Therapists often feel coerced into various transference-countertransference enactments that provide the patient with varying degrees of gratification of conscious or unconscious transference wishes. In a partial and attenuated way, therapists should allow themselves to be "sucked in" by the patient's interpersonal pressure (Hoffman and Gill 1988). Besides assisting the therapist in diagnosing the internal object world of the patient, the enactments may in and of themselves help the patient feel engaged with the therapist, held, and validated. The classical psychoanalytic posture of abstinence, objectivity, and anonymity may result in the patient's feeling abandoned. If Ms. Green's therapist had not increased his level of verbal activity and escalated his efforts to "pursue" her in response to her threats to flee the therapy, Ms. Green might well have experienced him as uncaring and discontinued therapy.

Transference interpretation must be used extremely judiciously in patients with histories of early trauma who externalize aggression.   The therapeutic alliance will suffer if externalized aggression is forced back down the patient's throat with transference interpretations. On the other hand, the alliance can be bolstered if the therapist empathically validates the patient's perspective in light of traumatic experiences in the past. Many children who are abused grow up with severely punitive and primitive superego formations. They engage in excessive self-blaming, assuming that the abuse they have suffered is deserved because of their essential badness. They often deal with their harsh superegos projectively by seeing others as attacking. Transference interpretations with such patients are experienced as critical attacks that are repetitions of early trauma, as illustrated by the responses of Ms. Green. On the other hand, a comment such as the following may help the patient feel understood: "I can understand why it might be difficult for you to trust me since in the past you have been terribly hurt and betrayed by people that you were supposed to be able to trust." A corollary of this point, in keeping with Epstein (1979) and Gabbard (1991), is that the therapist must hold and contain the "bad object" role for long periods of time until the patient opens up some degree of analytic space so that an interpretation can be considered in a meaningful way.

Transference interpretation may damage the therapeutic alliance in patients who are extremely narcissistically vulnerable and prone to feelings of shame and humiliation.   Narcissistically fragile patients often respond much better to expressions of affirmation or validation regarding the adaptive value of their defensive strategy. A sample intervention with such a patient might be worded as follows: "Given how badly you were hurt when your last relationship broke up, I can appreciate the logic of keeping distance from others for a while, including me." An interpretation that presents a view of the transference (or extratransference) situation that differs from the patient's objective experience will often be heard as tantamount to saying the patient is wrong, stupid, worthless, and so forth. One of the values of increased verbal activity with borderline patients is that they can hear the therapist's affirmation and validation of their internal experiences frequently in the course of a session. An example of this strategy that increased Ms. White's collaboration was her therapist's comment that "I think you're trying to face things in yourself and your life . . . more directly and more intensely than you have before."

The idealizing pole of a split transference may be internalized and lead to constructive changes.   Although splitting can be destructive to treatment in multiple-treater settings, therapists must recognize that it is unavoidable and necessary for the patient's emotional survival (Gabbard 1989). Although the ultimate goal is to integrate the positive and negative aspects of the self and object representations within the patient, the therapist who is uncomfortable in the idealized role and prematurely attempts to make the patient integrate disparate views of others is likely to damage the therapeutic alliance. As Kohut (1971) and Adler (1985) stressed, some patients need to idealize to repair a developmental deficit created by the absence of parental figures who could be idealized. A certain degree of tolerance of idealization, without engaging in devaluing and disparaging comments about other treaters who are in the bad object role, may promote internalizing processes, such as identification, that will ultimately strengthen the patient's ego and lead to a more durable self. This mechanism seemed particularly crucial to Ms. Green's improvement.

The patient's ability to collaborate with the therapist can be used as a within-session marker of how the therapy is progressing.   A corollary of this point, of course, is that when the collaboration deteriorates, the therapist and the patient should retrospectively examine what happened between them that made it more difficult for the patient to work with the therapist. Part of the examination should involve a willingness among therapists to examine their own role in the rupture, whether it be through countertransference, insensitivity, or errors in technique.

Positive transference and collaboration do not necessarily go hand in hand.   Although in some quarters the therapeutic alliance, or the concept of collaboration, is used interchangeably with Freud's notion of the unobjectionable positive transference, the two are not necessarily the same thing. In the case of Ms. Green, she perceived the therapist as warm, supportive, and helpful, but she found it difficult to collaborate with him in the service of working toward a consensually held therapeutic goal, because she could tolerate only mirroring and positively toned interventions. Our examination of the process data and the ratings suggests that Luborsky's distinction between Type I (experiencing the therapist as warm and helpful) and Type II (collaborating with the therapist) therapeutic alliances is valid and clinically useful.

Focusing on extratransference issues may paradoxically improve the patient's ability to work in the transference.   Therapists are often prone to attempt to bring the patient "kicking and screaming" into the transference when the patient is focusing primarily on extratransference issues. This strategy may be counterproductive in that borderline patients feel misunderstood and become more oppositional toward the therapist, thus damaging the therapeutic alliance. As illustrated in the vignette involving Ms. Green, empathic validation of the extratransference concerns and the patient's internal experience of the extratransference situation may ultimately result in the patient's increased ability to trust the therapist and work within the transference. A corollary of this point is that excessive transference interpretations may be counterproductive in therapeutic impasses.

Improved functioning should supersede the acquisition of insight as a therapeutic goal.   Contrary to conventional wisdom, some patients do not need greater insight to strengthen ego functioning necessary to lead a more productive life. Therapists of borderline patients must be diligent in separating out their own interests in interpretive work from the therapeutic needs of the patient. In some cases, insight may be necessary for the patient to progress in treatment and make significant strides in love and work outside the sessions. However, as the case of Ms. Green demonstrates, considerable gains are possible even though the patient's level of insight may be less after the treatment than before. This observation is in keeping with Wallerstein's (1986) and Horwitz's (1974) conclusions from their study of the PRP cases.

Maintaining professional boundaries makes effective psychotherapy possible.   A silent factor working behind the scenes with all three of our cases was the therapists' adherence to clear boundaries. Borderline patients typically coerce therapists out of their professional roles in a myriad of ways. Ms. Green, for example, referred to her previous therapist by his first name and viewed him as a friend who would supply her with drugs of abuse. Boundaries include considerations of such factors as role, time, place and space, money, gifts, language, self-disclosure, and physical contact (Gutheil and Gabbard 1993). Therapists should be diligent in monitoring deviations from standard practice in any of these areas as early warning signs of boundary diffusion and countertransference.

The ultimate message of this volume has been that therapists must adjust the treatment to the patient and not the patient to the treatment. There is inevitably a trial-and-error factor in the psychotherapy of borderline patients. To a large extent, the therapists who succeed are those who are willing to reassess their strategy repeatedly according to the shifting requirements of the patient within a particular session as well as across the course of therapy. A sense of the unpredictable and the unexpected lends an air of excitement and challenge to the treatment of these extraordinary patients.

References

Adler G: Borderline Psychopathology and Its Treatment. New York, Jason Aronson, 1985

Adler G: The myth of the therapeutic alliance with borderline patients revisited, in Handbook of Borderline Disorders. Edited by Silver D, Rosenbluth M. Madison, CT, International Universities Press, 1992, pp 251–267

Allen JG, Deering D, Buskirk JR, et al: Assessment of therapeutic alliances in the psychiatric hospital milieu. Psychiatry 51:291–299, 1988

American Psychiatric Association: Diagnostic and Statistical Manual of Mental Disorders, 3rd Edition, Revised. Washington, DC, American Psychiatric Association, 1987

Blatt SJ: Interpersonal relatedness and self-definition: two personality configurations and their implications for psychopathology and psychotherapy, in Repression and Dissociation: Implications for Personality Theory, Psychopathology and Health. Edited by Singer J. Chicago, IL, University of Chicago Press, 1990, pp 299–335

Blatt SJ: The differential effect of psychotherapy and psychoanalysis with anaclitic and introjective patients: the Menninger Psychotherapy Research Project revisited. J Am Psychoanal Assoc 40:691–724, 1992

Blatt SJ, Behrens RS: Separation-individuation, internalization and the nature of therapeutic action. Int J Psychoanal 68:279–297, 1987

Cooper AM: Psychic change: development in the theory of psychoanalytic techniques. Int J Psychoanal 73:245–250, 1992

Cornell DG, Silk KR, Ludolph PS, et al: Test-retest reliability of the Diagnostic Interview for Borderlines. Arch Gen Psychiatry 40:1307–1310, 1983

Crits-Christoph P, Barber JP, Krucias JS: The accuracy of therapists' interpretations and the development of the therapeutic alliance. Psychotherapy Research 3:25–35, 1993

Epstein L: Countertransference with borderline patients, in Countertransference. Edited by Epstein L, Feiner A. New York, Jason Aronson, 1979, pp 375–405

Frank AF: The therapeutic alliances of borderline patients, in Borderline Personality Disorder: Clinical and Empirical Perspectives. Edited by Clarkin JF, Marziali E, Munroe-Blum H. New York, Guilford, 1992, pp 220–247

Gabbard GO: Splitting in hospital treatment. Am J Psychiatry 146:444–451, 1989

Gabbard GO: Technical approaches to transference hate in the analysis of borderline patients. Int J Psychoanal 72:625–637, 1991

Gabbard GO: Psychodynamic Psychiatry in Clinical Practice: The DSM-IV Edition. Washington, DC, American Psychiatric Press, 1994

Gabbard GO, Wilkinson SM: The Management of Countertransference With Borderline Patients. Washington, DC, American Psychiatric Press, 1994

Gill MM: Analysis of Transference, Vol 1: Theory and Technique. New York, International Universities Press, 1982

Grinker RR Jr, Werble B, Drye RC: The Borderline Syndrome: A Behavioral Study of Ego Functions. New York, Basic Books, 1968

Gunderson JG: Borderline Personality Disorders. Washington, DC, American Psychiatric Press, 1984

Gunderson JG: Studies of borderline patients in psychotherapy, in Handbook of Borderline Disorders. Edited by Silver D, Rosenbluth M. Madison, CT, International Universities Press, 1992, pp 291–305

Gunderson J, Sabo AN: Treatment of borderline personality disorder: a critical review, in Borderline Personality Disorder: Etiology and Treatment. Edited by Paris J. Washington, DC, American Psychiatric Press, 1993, pp 385–406

Gunderson JG, Kolb JE, Austin V: The Diagnostic Interview for Borderline Patients. Am J Psychiatry 138:896–903, 1981

Gunderson J, Frank A, Ronningstam ER, et al: Early discontinuance of borderline patients from psychotherapy. J Nerv Ment Dis 177:38–42, 1989

Gutheil TG, Gabbard GO: The concept of boundaries in clinical practice: theoretical and risk-management dimensions. Am J Psychiatry 150:188–196, 1993

Hoffman IZ, Gill MM: Critical reflections on a coding scheme. Int J Psychoanal 69:55–64, 1988

Horwitz L: Clinical Prediction in Psychotherapy. New York, Jason Aronson, 1974

Kernberg OF: Severe Personality Disorders: Psychotherapeutic Strategies. New Haven, CT, Yale University Press, 1984

Kohut H: The Analysis of the Self. New York, International Universities Press, 1971

Luborsky L, Crits-Christoph P: Understanding Transference: The CCRT Method. New York, Basic Books, 1990

Meissner WW: The Borderline Spectrum: Differential Diagnosis and Developmental Issues. New York, Jason Aronson, 1984

Meissner WW: Treatment of Patients in the Borderline Spectrum. Northvale, NJ, Jason Aronson, 1988

Messer SB, Tishby O, Spillman A: Taking context seriously in psychotherapy research: relating therapist interventions to patient progress in brief psychodynamic therapy. J Consult Clin Psychol 60:678–688, 1992

Paris J, Zweig-Frank H: A critical review of the role of childhood sexual abuse in the etiology of borderline personality disorder. Can J Psychiatry 37:125–128, 1992

Pine F: The interpretive moment: variations on classical themes. Bull Menninger Clin 48:54–71, 1984

Piper WE, Azim HFA, Joyce AS, et al: Transference interpretations, therapeutic alliance, and outcome in short-term individual psychotherapy. Arch Gen Psychiatry 48:946–953, 1991

Piper WE, Azim HFA, Joyce AS, et al: Response to letter by Sigal. Arch Gen Psychiatry 50:1002, 1993

Pulver SE: Psychic change: insight or relationship? Int J Psychoanal 73:199–208, 1992

Rockland LH: Supportive Therapy for Borderline Patients. New York, Guilford, 1992

Sigal JJ: Transference interpretations, patients' gender, and dropout rates [letter]. Arch Gen Psychiatry 50:1002, 1993

Silberschatz G, Fretter PB, Curtis JT: How do interpretations influence the process of psychotherapy? J Consult Clin Psychol 54:646–652, 1986

Stone M: Etiology of borderline personality disorder: psychobiological factors contributing to an underlying irritability, in Borderline Personality Disorder: Etiology and Treatment. Edited by Paris J. Washington, DC, American Psychiatric Press, 1993, pp 87–101

Waldinger RJ, Gunderson JG: Effective Psychotherapy With Borderline Patients: Case Studies. New York, Macmillan, 1987

Wallerstein RS: Forty-two Lives in Treatment: A Study of Psychoanalysis and Psychotherapy. New York, Guilford, 1986

Weiss J: How Psychotherapy Works: Process and Technique. New York, Guilford, 1993

Zanarini MC, Gunderson JG, Marino MF, et al: Childhood experiences of borderline patients. Compr Psychiatry 30:18–25, 1989

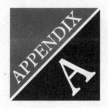

Chapter Notes

Mr. Black

1. Over a period of several months, the intervention and thera-peutic alliance subgroups met to rate a total of 17 transcribed sessions from the psychotherapy of Mr. Black. The sessions chosen ranged from session 16 to session 728. Either two or three consecutive sessions were chosen from different points in the treatment.

As described earlier, each week the two subgroups would rate the same session and then meet to assess the linkage of the therapist's interventions with the patient's shifts in collaboration. After the therapeutic alliance subgroup shared with the other subgroup the lo-cations within each session of the shifts in collaboration, each of the six researchers would individually write out a narrative for each shift and identify which interventions, if any, contributed to the shift in collaboration. The six researchers would then share their observations and reach a consensus about the factors that were most likely to have influenced the shift.

As Appendix D, Table D–3 demonstrates, of a total of 17 sessions, 48 shifts in collaboration were identified by the therapeutic alliance subgroup. The shifts per session ranged from 1 to 6, with a mean of 2.8. Of the 48 shifts, 36 could be clearly related to the therapist's in-terventions.

2.   Mr. Black's increased alliance with the therapist was not reflected in the patient's overall collaboration ratings. Rather, all the overall collaboration scores on our 5-point scale for the 17 sessions, with the exception of the last, were monotonously uniform and wavered between 3.5 and 4. In the very last session, he attained a rating of 4.5. Our explanation for this finding has partly to do with the patient's personality organization and partly with a characteristic of our scale. As noted earlier, the patient was a highly obsessional, intellectualizing man who tended to keep his affects under tight control and rarely permitted himself to display intense feelings. Hence, changes in his collaboration were rather difficult to discern.

In addition, we believe that the scale itself was not as sensitive as it might have been to significant changes, particularly for higher-functioning patients such as Mr. Black. He started at a relatively high level of our scale, and the narrow range for improvement was a limiting factor. This consideration is somewhat bolstered by the fact that the Luborsky Helping Alliance ratings, a 7-point scale, did show a small, but suggestive increase during the latter third of the treatment (i.e., sessions 527–728). On the one hand, the sessions up to 526 stayed in the range from 4.5 to 6, whereas after session 256, the range was 5.5–7. These were the scores on Type 1, which reflects a positive bonding with the therapist, as opposed to Type 2, which assesses the patient's perception of working in tandem with the therapist.

3.   During the first half of the treatment, until session 404, the ratio of transference interventions (R) compared with nontransference interventions (X) was clearly in favor of transference by an average of about 2:1 (see Appendix D, Table D–2). Beginning with session 405, the tilt was in the opposite direction, with the nontransference interventions predominating also by a ratio of 2:1. Did this mean that a shift occurred midway in the treatment from expressive to supportive? The research team's ratings on our Supportive-Expressive Scale show no indication of such a shift. Rather, an expressiveness score of 5–6 on a 7-point scale was fairly consistent throughout the treatment, whereas the supportiveness rating stayed at a 2–3 level.

This observation underscores the fact that a highly expressive treatment is not necessarily and exclusively a transference-focused treatment. Clearly, extratransference interventions can be quite powerful in improving the therapeutic alliance. The researchers also noted a substantial increase in the number of affirmations (Appendix D, Table D–2) in the second half of the treatment. This increase may correlate well with the predominance of X ratings over R ratings in the latter of part of the therapy. We believe that the patient began to work on the transference on his own, requiring fewer interpretations by the therapist.

Ms. Green

4. Of a total of 18 sessions, 32 shifts in collaboration were identified by the therapeutic alliance subgroup (see Appendix D, Table D–7). The number of shifts per session ranged from 0 to 4, with a mean of 1.7. Of the 32 shifts, 25 could be clearly related to interventions by the therapist. In some cases, one intervention immediately preceding the shift was clearly causal. But in most instances, a series of interventions seemed to culminate in a change in collaboration. Still other shifts seemed to stem from the therapeutic climate established by the therapist's perseverance and empathic or encouraging comments throughout the session. On one occasion, a shift seemed to occur relatively spontaneously.

5. Ms. Green's average level of collaboration over the course of psychotherapy was 2.7 on a 7-point scale, between "significant limitations to collaboration" (3.0) and "the concept of collaboration hardly applies" (2.0). At best, in 3 of the 18 sessions we studied, her collaboration was 3.5 (between "significant limitations" and "periodic interruptions" of collaboration). Although varying from session to session, her overall collaboration tended to deteriorate over the course of the therapy (first third, 3.0; second third, 2.6; final third, 2.4). Notably, within sessions (comparing first and last thirds of each session), Ms. Green, on average, showed no improvement in collaboration.

The relatively low level of collaboration and the declining trend of collaboration across therapy were reflected in both components of collaboration that we measured; namely, the extent to which Ms. Green made use of the therapist's interventions and the degree to which she brought in significant issues. Of particular significance is that our collaboration scale is weighted toward an expressive, insight-oriented approach, inasmuch as the optimal level of collaboration entails bringing in significant issues, working actively and reflectively with the material that emerges, applying insights, and analyzing resistances rather than acting them out. This is precisely the kind of work to which Ms. Green showed an aversion.

Ms. White

6.   We evaluated a total of 18 sessions, ranging from session 6 through session 144, with three consecutive sessions chosen at each of six different points in the treatment. The procedure the judges followed is noted in Appendix B (pp. 189–190). A total of 26 shifts in collaboration were identified. The number of shifts in each session ranged from 0 to 2, with an average 1.4. Of the 26 shifts, 21 were clearly related to the therapist's interventions.

7.   The consistent pattern that Ms. White demonstrated throughout the course of the 2-year psychotherapy was to deepen her level of collaboration within each session. Of the 18 sessions rated, 12 reflected an improvement in collaboration when comparing the last third of the session with the first third. In only one session was there a lower collaboration rating at the end. The great majority of the shifts in collaboration occurred in the second and last thirds of each of those sessions, whereas the overall level of collaboration remained high throughout, as reflected, for example, in the Luborsky Type I and Type II ratings. Overall, the Luborsky Type I ratings ranged from a low of 4 to a high of 9, with a preponderance of scores clustering around 7. There was a slight dip midway through the treatment process into the 5–6 range that persisted through a significant portion of the middle phase of treatment, with a sharp resurgence in the latter third of the treatment, reflecting a significant increase in the positive bonding with the therapist. There was not, however, a similar pattern observed for Type II, which reflects the patient's perception of working in tandem with the therapist. There, the scores remained consistently in the 5–7 range, a finding basically in keeping with our assessment of the overall level of collaboration.

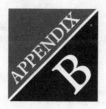

Instruments

Therapeutic Alliance: Patient Collaboration

Rationale

There is a broad consensus in the field of psychotherapy and psychotherapy research that establishing a good therapeutic alliance is a cornerstone of psychotherapy, and this conviction has been supported amply by research (Frieswyk et al. 1986). In a survey of the 100-year history of psychotherapy, Freedheim et al. (1992) concluded that the therapeutic alliance is one of a handful of major themes. Research on outcome of psychotherapy has consistently attested to the effectiveness of a variety of approaches, underscoring the universal significance of "common factors," among which the therapeutic alliance is prominent. The therapeutic alliance is particularly critical in the treatment of borderline patients because of the intense, unstable, and distrustful nature of their relationships. In fact, the major challenge in treating these patients is to find a way to establish a productive alliance. As Frieswyk et al. (1986) put it, "The development of the alliance is at the center of the treatment for the borderline patient. Its success or failure and its vicissitudes spell the outcome of the process" (p. 37).

Definition

Research on the therapeutic alliance has been characterized by a wide range of conceptualizations and definitions of the alliance. Most im-

187

portantly, for those interested in studying therapist technique, the study of the alliance has been confounded by combining contributions of both patient and therapist in the conceptualization of the alliance.

To study the impact of therapist technique on the alliance, we have chosen to focus on one facet of the alliance, namely, the patient's collaboration in the process. We conceptualized the patient's collaboration as the extent to which the patient makes optimal use of the therapy as a resource for constructive change (Frieswyk et al. 1984). We also developed a scale to measure patients' collaboration that could be rated with adequate interrater reliability (Allen et al. 1984).

Our initial assessments of patient collaboration were conducted at a relatively global level; that is, raters assessed the patient's collaboration for a whole psychotherapy session (i.e., rating overall collaboration for the session). This type of assessment is appropriate for tracking collaboration over the course of an entire psychotherapy process or for examining collaboration at a particular phase of psychotherapy.

For the purposes of studying the impact of therapist interventions on collaboration, however, we needed a more molecular measure of collaboration. In developing molecular measures, we adopted the approach advocated by Rice and Greenberg (1984): "The intense scrutiny of particular classes of recurrent change episodes in psychotherapy, making fine-grained descriptions of these moments of change together with the patterns of client-therapist interactions that form their context" (p. 13). That is, we focused on *shifts* in the patient's collaboration that occurred *within* psychotherapy hours. We defined upward shifts as follows. "In comparison with the previous segment: The patient introduces particularly significant material, becomes more reflective about the material, begins to explore and examine resistance rather than enacting it, or makes better use of the therapist's interventions." In contrast, we defined a downward shift as follows. "In comparison with the previous segment: The patient moves away from significant issues (e.g., changing to a more neutral topic or intellectualizing), becomes less reflective (e.g., begins externalizing), begins to give in to resistance rather than analyzing it, or makes less use of the therapist's interventions (e.g., ignores or defeats them)." These general definitions have been supplemented in a rating manual with detailed clinical vignettes illustrating upward and downward shifts, numerous other examples, and rating conventions.

As we studied sessions in-depth with the goal of detecting changes, we observed more gradual changes within sessions in addition to the more abrupt shifts. We have called these gradual changes "drifts" (Allen et al. 1990). Specifically, we were able to use our global collaboration scale (Allen et al. 1984) to rate thirds of sessions (i.e., first, second, and third parts). Moreover, based on a previous study (Allen et al. 1984), we distinguished two key components of collaboration: the extent to which the patient is *addressing significant issues* and the extent to which the patient is *making use of the therapist's interventions.* Like the global collaboration scale, gradual changes within sessions (drifts from one third to the next) could feasibly be assessed in the extent to which the patient was bringing up significant issues and the extent to which the patient was making good use of the therapist's interventions.

To supplement our own measures of collaboration, we also employed Luborsky et al.'s (1983) well-established measure of the therapeutic alliance that consists of global ratings of an entire session. Luborsky et al. have distinguished two facets of the alliance: Type 1, "in which the patient experiences the therapist as providing, or being capable of providing, the help which is needed" (p. 481), and Type 2, "in which the patient experiences treatment as a process of working together with the therapist toward the goals of the treatment" (p. 481). There are six subscales of the Type 1 alliance and four subscales of the Type 2 alliance; ratings for each type are averages across the subscales.

Procedures

Typed transcripts of each psychotherapy session were independently evaluated by the three members of the patient-collaboration subgroup. To avoid confounding the ratings of our own measures of the alliance (i.e., shifts and collaboration) with the measures developed by Luborsky, the Luborsky alliance scales were rated by the other subgroup of raters who categorized the therapist interventions.

For each transcript of each session, the raters independently made several ratings. First, for 50-line segments of transcript, raters indicated whether there was an upward shift, a downward shift, or no shift. We had originally divided positive and negative ratings into possible shift versus clear shift, but we were unable to make such a fine discrimination and collapsed the ratings into upward or downward shifts. Second, for thirds of each session, raters assessed collaboration, extent of significant issues, and use of therapist interventions. Third, for each session, raters also assessed overall collaboration across the entire session. Fourth, as previously stated, the Luborsky Helping Alliance Scales were rated by another team of raters when they rated the therapist interventions.

After the three raters had independently rated the collaboration scales (i.e., shifts, thirds of sessions, overall ratings), they compared the ratings and obtained a consensus score. We identified for further study only those shifts that were observed by at least two of the three raters.

Reliability

The reliability of our global collaboration scale had been established in a previous study (Allen et al. 1984). Assessment of our more molecular measures, however, required additional research, the results of which have been presented in detail elsewhere (Allen et al. 1990) and are briefly summarized here. The raters for this previous reliability study were the same as those in the subgroup who assessed the transcripts for the current research; they rated transcripts of an individual session for 39 separate patients, rating 411 fifty-line segments of transcript in all. We found that we could assess drifts across thirds of sessions (significant issues and use of interventions) with generally adequate reliability, although our reliability was higher on one series of cases than another (Spearman-Brown corrected coefficients for "issues" ranging from .69 to .81 for one series and from .53 to .64 for the other, and for "use" ranging from .67 to .83 for one series and from .45 to .58 for the other).

Obtaining reliable ratings of shifts in collaboration proved to be relatively problematic, in part owing to the low base rate of shifts within sessions. For the majority of the segments (55%), no rater detected a shift. Kappa coefficients were uniformly low and not statistically significant. Tabulation and visual inspection of the data revealed a sizable proportion of idiosyncratic ratings; that is, only one rater rated a shift for 26% of the total segments. Thus, for 26% of the segments rated, the raters reached no agreement that a shift occurred. However, an obvious clustering of shift ratings occurred at various junctures across the series of cases, even though such occurrences were relatively infrequent. Two or three raters agreed that shifts occurred in 78 (19%) of the segments, which approximates the base rate for shifts. For 66 of these 78 segments (85%) in which more than one rater detected a shift, the raters attained complete agreement about the direction of the shift. There was unanimous agreement on the occurrence and direction of 19 shifts.

We computed comparable statistics to the reliability study just described for the three patients in the current study, finding roughly the same pattern of agreement (Table B–1). From ratings of 435 segments across the three patients, we found that there was complete agreement on "no shift" for 44%. This is somewhat lower than the 55% figure for the reliability study, suggesting that the raters may have lowered their threshold somewhat for detecting shifts. For 28% of the segments, only one of the three raters detected a shift; these were considered idiosyncratic ratings (comparable to the 26% in the reliability study). Two or three raters agreed that shifts occurred in 28% of the segments (somewhat higher than the 19% agreement in the reliability study), and when more than one rater detected a shift, they agreed on the direction of the shift in 76% of the cases (slightly lower than the 86% figure in the reliability study). There was unanimous agreement on the occurrence and direction of 37 shifts.

We were dismayed that we had taken great pains to conceptualize and operationalize shifts in collaboration and nevertheless had such

Table B–1. Reliability of patient collaboration ratings

	Intraclass correlations average
Shifts within session (upward or downward)	Low
Drifts within session (rating of each third)	.66
Collaboration level (overall)	.69
Luborsky Helping Alliance (overall)	
Type I	.83
Type II	.72

difficulty obtaining independent agreement. One would expect like-minded clinicians to agree on a phenomenon of seemingly obvious significance in the psychotherapy process. Accepting that assessments of patient shifts in collaboration during the hours are more elusive than we would have thought, we adopted a consensus method of identifying shifts. Although we spelled out the rationale for this approach previously, we list it here again for convenience.

> We are searching for an event with a relatively low base rate, and we are attempting to make relatively sophisticated clinical judgments. We agree with Rice and Greenberg's [1984] contention that "the best instrument for pattern identification [is] the 'human integrator,' who in psychotherapy research would be the disciplined clinical observer" (p. vi). At the level of ordinary clinical concepts, there is no way around clinical judgment with inevitable individual differences in perception and interpretation.
>
> In searching for clinically significant events, the best hedge against idiosyncratic results is reliance on the agreement of a number of expert judges who have made independent observations. Inspection of our raw data led us to adopt a "consensus" method of selecting only those shifts for which there was independent agreement between at least two of three raters (and no disagreement about direction). Reliance on such convergence of independent opinions provides some assurance that only the most detectable instances of shifts will be selected for subsequent research scrutiny. (Allen et al. 1990, p. 527)

Therapist Interventions

Rationale

In an early phase of our research planning, the investigators studied the content of therapy sessions and reviewed existing systems for scoring content within therapy hours (Gill and Hoffman 1982; Kernberg 1983; Luborsky 1976; Strupp 1980). This search was guided by several goals: 1) to find a means of differentiating between transference versus nontransference interventions, 2) to assess transference versus nontransference interpretations, and 3) to assess the various forms of intervention that might precede and culminate in transference-focused comments. Gill and Hoffman's (1982) system was most compatible with these interests because of the advantages posed by their attention to transference versus nontransference patient content and interpretive versus noninterpretive interventions. As we began applying Gill and Hoffman's "process coding categories" to typed transcripts of psychotherapy hours, we discovered some interesting links between transference work and overall therapeutic alliance ratings (Gabbard et al. 1988; Horwitz and Frieswyk 1980), but we also encountered some limitations in the intervention categories. Following our early exploratory work, we continued to modify and simplify Gill and Hoffman's system. The system we used of rating each intervention in the session is a simplified version of Gill and Hoffman's system and includes a reduced number of intervention categories. Coincident with the development of our category system, Marziali (1984) used a similar system to predict outcome of brief psychotherapy. However, our method has the advantages of including 12 categories rather than Marziali's three, allowing a more detailed examination of the breadth and variety of supportive and expressive work and the work done by the therapist to prepare for interpretation.

Definition

Each therapist intervention was assigned two scores. The first score indicates one of six types of intervention: interpretation (I), confrontation (C), clarification (CL), encouragement to elaborate (E), empathic (EM), and advice and praise (AP). An additional category was used to denote simple affirmations ("yes," "uh huh") by the therapist (A). The second score accompanies each of the six categories and indicates whether the intervention is addressed to the patient-therapist relationship or transference (R) versus matters outside the relationship (X). The six major types of intervention, each scored for transference versus nontransference focus, plus the A category, constitute a total of 13 scoring categories (see Appendix E, pp. 243–244).

Because interventions vary in effectiveness depending on the skill with which they are formulated and stated, the raters also developed a 6-point scale to rate competence of the interventions that was completed for each intervention and for the overall session. However, there was such a narrow range of the competence ratings, primarily in the direction of high competence, that the data were not used in our analysis.

Procedures

The three raters independently scored each therapist intervention for a given session. Then they met to discuss the scores and arrived at a consensus score for each intervention.

Reliability

Similar to the reliability of our therapeutic alliance scale, interrater agreement for the therapist intervention categories was assessed in a prior research project by comparing three raters' scores of typed transcripts of single therapy hours for 39 different patients. For all sessions, the raters scored every therapist intervention.

In the early study, we attempted to establish interrater reliability. The three raters independently scored the first 20 cases, then paused to discuss scoring discrepancies and slightly modified the scoring criteria in the hope of improving reliability for a second set of 19 cases. Thus, the data consisted of two successive samples. The scoring was guided by a detailed manual of instructions with examples.

To ensure the generalizability of our category system, we obtained transcripts for long- and short-term psychotherapies and from three different centers for psychotherapy research. Drs. Lester Luborsky (the Penn Psychotherapy Project) and Hans Strupp (the Vanderbilt Project) sent us typed transcripts from their psychotherapy research samples, and in addition, we solicited transcripts from Menninger Clinic psychotherapists. All patients were considered by their respective therapist to fall into the category of borderline personality disorder.

An overview of these findings is as follows. The reliabilities for each of the 12 intervention categories (assessed category by category across thirds of sessions) were inconsistent, and many did not reach acceptable levels. We also examined several other forms of reliability, finding that reliabilities were good for the total number of each scoring category in a session, for the categories representing a continuum from least expressive (advice and praise) to most (interpretation), for the transference (R) versus nontransference (X) focus of interventions, and for the degree of supportiveness or expressiveness scales (to be described below).

A reliability analysis that was fairly successful employed intraclass correlations, with the Spearman-Brown correction (r_k), for the total number of each scoring category in a session. We considered r_k's of .60–.69 as borderline and .70 or better as acceptable. In the first series, 9 of 13 reliabilities (69%) were at an acceptable or better level, and 2 were borderline; for the second series, 10 of 13 categories (77%) were at an acceptable level. For 2 of our unreliable categories in the first series and 3 in the second, frequency of those particular interventions was so low that an assessment of reliability was limited. For the majority of categories there are statistically significant mean level differences among the three raters, suggesting the need for at least two raters to control for such rater bias. Because we were interested in the relationship between individual interventions and shifts in collaboration, we used consensus scores in our data analysis.

We considered our intervention categories, excluding the X versus R distinction, as a continuum from supportive to expressive types of interventions. The order was as follows: advice and praise (AP), empathic (EM), encouragement to elaborate (E), clarification (CL), confrontation (C), and interpretation (I). We calculated the interrater agreement on these continuum scores for the first intervention in each third of a session scored by all three raters. Of the 6 intraclass correlations, 5 (83%) were at a better than acceptable level, with the 1 remaining correlation falling in the marginally acceptable range (.64).

The investigators also assessed the reliability of judgments about whether interventions are focused on transference (therapy relationship) or nontransference (nonrelationship) using the previously described R versus X scores. The statistical analysis appropriate to such category data is Cohen's kappa, the percentage of agreement corrected for chance of each rater paired with each other. We attempted to select the first intervention in each third of the session scored by all three raters for reliability assessment, but the frequency of occurrence of interventions about the therapy relationship for the first third was inadequate. For the first series, all of the kappas exceeded an acceptable level, which we considered as .40 or better. For the second series, 5 of 6 of the kappas (83%) were at an acceptable or better level, with the remaining kappa at a marginally acceptable level. Reliabilities tended to be greater in the last third of the sessions, likely because transference interventions were made with the greatest frequency in the latter part of the therapy sessions.

After scoring the first series of 20 cases, the raters decided to add a measure of the degree of supportiveness and expressiveness of the therapy sessions. Consequently, we devised two 5-point rating scales that were used to rate the second series.

The scales for supportiveness and expressiveness were applied only to the second series of 19 cases. The corrected intraclass reliabilities expressed the agreement among our three raters for the sessions divided into thirds. We also rated the overall session on these two scales. Both expressive and supportive scales were at marginally acceptable levels for the first third of the sessions, when the therapists tended to be less active, and all the remaining reliabilities were consistently at better than acceptable levels (between .73 and .84).

Finally, we examined the intercorrelations among the various measures of supportiveness versus expressiveness: namely, the continuum, the X versus R distinction, and the expressiveness and supportiveness scales (Table B–2). The expectable significant correlations between X versus R and the latter two scales emerge, particularly in the last two thirds of the sessions.

Once the main study was concluded, we wished to compare the results of the initial reliability study, previously described, with interrater agreement among the therapist intervention raters for the three cases in the present study. We computed the percentage of agree-

Table B–2. Reliability of intervention ratings

	Intraclass correlations average
Single scores	Low
Total scores/session	.69
Continuum: expressive → supportive	.80
Relationship versus nonrelationship	.68
Competence of interventions	.70
Expressiveness and supportiveness scales 7-point scales, overall	.78

ment among raters for each case on various selected intervention categories. If one views 70% as an adequate percentage of agreement and 60%–69% as marginal agreement, the results show variability in reliability for the categories. The category encouragement to elaborate (E) reached fairly good agreement, interpretation (I) was marginally adequate, whereas clarification (CL) and confrontation (C) failed to reach acceptable levels of agreement. The distinction of transference focus (R) versus nontransference focus (X), for the most part, fell in the marginally adequate to adequate range.

Linking Patient Collaboration to Therapist Interventions

As previously described, we developed a method that would enable us to assess shifts in the patient's collaboration associated with specific therapeutic interventions. The research team rated and studied each case in succession (Mr. Black, Ms. Green, then Ms. White), proceeding session by session for each case. For each session, three members assessed collaboration, and three other members assessed interventions. After each subgroup reached consensus, the consensus ratings for the session were distributed to the whole six-member group (i.e., each member knew where upward and downward shifts had been pinpointed and how each intervention was categorized). Then each member independently wrote down a judgment about the link between shifts in collaboration and the prior interventions. These independent assessments were then distributed among the research team members and discussed with the goal of developing a consensus regarding the link between each collaboration shift and preceding events. Thus, the final product was a determination of relationships among interventions and shifts in collaboration and a clinical conceptualization of the possible reasons for those shifts or lack of shifts.

Predictions

Rationale

The research was designed to examine hypotheses about the optimal therapeutic strategy for treating various kinds of borderline patients.

We hoped to contribute to a delineation of patient characteristics that would reflect amenability to a more supportive versus a more expressive treatment approach. Although we had certain exclusion criteria, we did not specify in advance any characteristics beyond meeting criteria for borderline personality disorder.

We developed a prediction component of the study to serve two functions: 1) to provide a comprehensive assessment of patient characteristics that we considered likely to bear on suitability for expressive or supportive approaches and 2) to provide a priori predictions of the optimal (supportive or expressive) approach on the basis of the comprehensive assessment to confirm or disconfirm commonly held assumptions regarding the treatment of borderline patients.

Procedures

Each of the two prediction raters was given the following clinical material: initial case summary, family history, psychological test report, videotape of the initial Diagnostic Interview for Borderline Patients (DIB) (Gunderson et al. 1981) interview, transcripts of three early psychotherapy sessions, and ratings of the Bellak Scales of Ego Functions (Bellak and Goldsmith 1973) (the latter supplied by another pair of raters). For each of the three patients, the raters independently reviewed the clinical material and made their ratings. Having arrived at the ratings independently, they jointly reviewed each rating, arrived at a consensus score for the quantitative ratings, and arrived at a consensus narrative for each qualitative assessment (i.e., a consensus answer to each question).

Variables

Patient characteristics.　The comprehensive assessment of patient characteristics consisted of two parts: one quantitative and the other qualitative. First, raters assessed each patient on the following 10-point scales: friendliness, likability, intelligence, motivation, psychological-mindedness, conscience factors, self-discipline, impulse control, defensive style, externalization/internalization, empathy/narcissism, parental factors, and social supports (see Appendix E, Prediction Study Manual).

Second, raters provided a qualitative description of the patient's pattern of relationships, focusing on closeness-seeking or distance-taking behavior with regard to significant others. Raters addressed four questions: To what extent does the patient strive for and achieve a mature emotional closeness to significant others in which appropriate boundaries are maintained between self and others? To what extent does the patient strive for and maintain symbiotic-merger relations with significant others, including attention to patient's dependency wishes, magical expectations, and separation reactions? To what extent does the patient strive for and maintain emotional distance from significant others? To what extent does the patient fluctuate between a position of closeness and emotional relatedness on the one hand and withdrawal and distance on the other?

Optimal therapeutic strategy. On the basis of their assessments of these patient characteristics, raters predicted the optimal therapeutic strategy, with attention to the extent to which the treatment should be supportive or expressive. These judgments also included quantitative ratings and qualitative assessments. Having been given definitions of supportiveness and expressiveness (see Appendix E, Prediction Study Manual), raters indicated on two 7-point scales the extent to which expressive techniques and supportive techniques should be used. Independent scales were employed because of the conviction that supportive and expressive approaches are not necessarily antithetical (i.e., a treatment process could include both supportive and expressive interventions). In addition, raters indicated on two 7-point scales the optimal degree of focus on patient-therapist relationship (from no emphasis to great emphasis) and the optimal degree of focus on nonrelationship matters (none to great).

In addition to these quantitative ratings, judges made qualitative assessments in addressing several questions pertaining to the main therapeutic issues anticipated, the issues that should be addressed by expressive-uncovering techniques, the issues that should be addressed by supportive techniques, anticipated shifts in treatment approaches during the course of therapy, and patient characteristics bearing on the predictions made.

Intervention profile. Judges were asked to forecast the optimal treatment approach by making quantitative and qualitative determinations about the relative use of the range of therapist interventions conceptualized by the research team. That is, they rated the extent to which each of the following types of therapist interventions should be emphasized (using 7-point scales ranging from no emphasis to great emphasis): interpretation, confrontation, clarification, encouragement to elaborate, affirmation, empathy, and advice-praise. In addition to these quantitative ratings, judges described qualitatively the degree of emphasis on each type of intervention they thought optimal and their reason for their judgment.

Outcome Assessment

Rationale

The long-standing debate between process-oriented and outcome-oriented approaches to psychotherapy research appears to be moving toward a resolution embodied in the consensus that the two approaches should be combined—that is, to "emphasize specifically the relation between process and outcome" (Beutler et al. 1991, p. 326). Our examination of the relation between interventions and patient collaboration is consistent with this thrust. That is, shifts in collaboration can be construed as "sub-outcomes," described by Safran et al. (1988, p. 5) as being "linked together on the pathway toward ultimate outcome" (see Allen et al. 1990). More generally, we have construed the patient's collaboration as "the final common pathway for a host of therapist and patient contributions" and, therefore, "a marker of the effectiveness of the therapy process" (Colson et al. 1988, p. 264). Yet, to evaluate the impact of the therapeutic strategy, we also assessed outcome in the traditional sense, using a comprehensive evaluation of the patient's functioning at termination and follow-up as contrasted with functioning at the time of beginning treatment.

Procedures

For their initial ratings, the two outcome raters were provided with the following material: case summary, family history, psychological test report, initial DIB interview, and transcripts of the first three sessions. For their posttreatment ratings, they were provided with the following material: discharge summary, termination psychological test report, termination DIB interview, and transcripts of the last three psychotherapy sessions. The judges made all assessments independently, and then they conferred to arrive at consensus ratings for the quantitative variables and a consensus narrative for the qualitative evaluations.

Variables

Initial. The judges rated each patient on the Global Assessment Scale (Endicott et al. 1976), four 7-point Levels of Functioning Scales (ego function, behavior, object relations, and sense of self), and 10 Ego Functions Scales (reality testing, judgment, regulation and control, object relations, thought processes, defensive functioning, autonomous functioning, synthetic-integrative functioning, mastery-competence, and superego adaptation) (Bellak and Goldsmith 1973). In addition, the judges described each of the following patient characteristics in a paragraph: core neurotic conflicts, self-concept, insight, psychological-mindedness, and transference paradigms.

Posttreatment. Judges rated each patient by using the same scales as during the initial assessment, namely, global assessment of functioning, level of function, and ego functions. In addition, they described in narrative form the *change* in the following: core neurotic conflicts, self-concept, insight, psychological-mindedness, and transference paradigms. They also made a qualitative assessment of the patient characteristics that they judged to be most influential in the outcome of treatment.

References

Allen J, Newsom G, Gabbard GO, et al: Scales to assess the therapeutic alliance from a psychoanalytic perspective. Bull Menninger Clin 48:383–400, 1984

Allen J, Gabbard GO, Newsom GE, et al: Detecting patterns of change in patients' collaboration within individual psychotherapy sessions. Psychotherapy 27:522–530, 1990

Bellak L, Goldsmith L: The Broad Scope of Ego Function Assessment. New York, Wiley, 1973

Beutler LE, Crago M, Machado PPP: The status of programmatic research, in Psychotherapy Research. Edited by Beutler LE, Crago M. Washington, DC, American Psychological Press, 1991, pp 325–328

Colson DB, Horwitz L, Allen JG, et al: Patient collaboration as a criterion for the therapeutic alliance. Psychoanalytic Psychology 5:259–268, 1988

Endicott J, Spitzer R, Fleiss, J, et al: The Global Assessment Scale. Arch Gen Psychiatry 33:766–771, 1976

Freedheim DK, Freudenberger HJ, Kessler JW, et al (eds): History of Psychotherapy: A Century of Change. Washington, DC, American Psychological Association, 1992

Frieswyk SH, Colson DB, Allen JG: Conceptualizing the therapeutic alliance from a psychoanalytic perspective. Psychotherapy 21:460–464, 1984

Frieswyk SH, Allen JG, Colson DB, et al: The therapeutic alliance: its place as a process and outcome variable in psychotherapy research. J Consult Clin Psychol 54:32–38, 1986

Gabbard GO, Horwitz L, Frieswyk SH, et al: The effect of therapist interventions on the therapeutic alliance with borderline patients. J Am Psychoanal Assoc 36:697–727, 1988

Gill MM, Hoffman I: A method for studying the analysis of aspects of the patient's experience of the relationship in psychoanalysis and psychotherapy. J Am Psychoanal Assoc 30:137–167, 1982

Gunderson JG, Kolb JE, Austin V: The Diagnostic Interview for Borderline Patients. Am J Psychiatry 138:896–903, 1981

Horwitz L, Frieswyk S: The impact of interpretation on therapeutic alliance in borderline patients. Paper presented at the meeting of the American Psychoanalytic Association, New York, December 1980

Kernberg OF: From the Menninger project to a research strategy for long term psychotherapy of borderline personality disorders, in Psychotherapy Research: Where Are We and Where Shall We Go? Edited by Williams JB, Spitzer RL. New York, Guilford, 1983, pp 247–260

Luborsky L: Helping alliance in psychotherapy, in Successful Psychotherapy. Edited by Claghorn JL. New York, Brunner/Mazel, 1976, pp 92–116

Luborsky L, Crits-Christoph P, Alexander L, et al: Two helping alliance methods for predicting outcomes of psychotherapy. J Nerv Ment Dis 17:480–491, 1983

Marziali EA: Prediction of outcome of brief psychotherapy from therapist interpretive interventions. Arch Gen Psychiatry 41:301–304, 1984

Rice LH, Greenberg L (eds): Patterns of Change. New York, Guilford, 1984
Safran J, Greenberg LS, Rice LN: Integrating psychotherapy research and
    practice: modeling the change process. Psychotherapy 25:1–17, 1988
Strupp HH: Success and failure in time-limited psychotherapy. Arch Gen
    Psychiatry 37:595–603, 1980

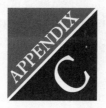

Log Linear Analysis

I t was anticipated originally that the data collected in this study would be time-series data. As the study evolved, it became apparent that a continuous unbroken series of timed observations could not be collected. For Mr. Black, a quasi-random selection of sessions to be transcribed and rated resulted in 17 sessions, of which 6 were sequential pairs and 1 was a sequential triplet, but there were big time lapses between the pairs, triplets, or individual sessions. Ms. Green and Ms. White had 6 triplets of successive sessions, but the triplets were separated in time. Within a session, time, as such, was not a unit; rather, number of lines in the typed transcript became a proxy for a time interval. However, there were differences within and (particularly) between patients in the number of lines per session so that a uniform unit could not be assumed. Some kind of statistical analysis was desired that would link therapy interventions and shifts in the patient's collaboration in a way that took account of a particular intervention occurring before a particular shift in the collaboration. Roger Bakeman's sequential analysis method using log linear analysis (Bakeman 1978, 1983; Bakeman and Gottman 1986) seemed to fit our requirements.

Method

With this sequential analysis, the data can be sequential event data, timed sequential data, or timed sequential event data. We conceptualized our data as sequential event data; that is, shifts in the collaboration comprised a sequence of coded events, coded in four categories: positive shift, positive partial shift, negative partial shift, and negative shift. The second sequence of events was that of intervention; each type of intervention coded present or absent was considered as an event sequence. The reliability of the coding of these two sets of events has been addressed in Appendix B (Tables B–1 and B–2). The basic descriptive statistics are counts or proportions for each kind of event considered separately or jointly. The first level of analysis of such count data involves tabulating the sequential data into frequency or contingency tables. Bakeman developed his sequential analysis approach with interaction data, in which a participant behaves in a certain way (antecedent event) and a second participant responds in a certain way (consequent event). The sequential nature of the data is captured by the notion of lag; the first observation is lag 0, the next lag 1, the next lag 2, and so on. If interest is in adjacent relationships, a contingency table would compare lag 0 (antecedent) with lag 1 (consequent), and the frequencies in this table would be tallied across a series of observations. In our data, the antecedent event is a particular therapeutic intervention, and a shift in the collaboration is the consequent event. Only lag 0 to lag 1 (i.e., adjacent) relationships are of interest. Other categorized events can also be included by the use of multidimensional contingency tables. Not all dimensions in a contingency table need to refer to lag positions; they can be other independent categorized events. Bakeman, in a personal consultation, felt that combining observations over sessions, even though they were not in sequence, would not invalidate the method. We would be asking the question, "Does event 1 (presence of a particular intervention) precede event 2 (a shift in the collaboration)?" over a series of observations where the series includes both observations within sessions and across sessions. In our study, an additional event was block: that is, sessions categorized into early, middle, and late. Since these categories were quite separated in time, the assumption of relative independence is not untenable.

Given two-dimensional (or more) contingency tables, hierarchical log linear analysis (Bishop et al. 1975) can be used to answer questions concerning the significance of an individual dimension (event) or the interaction of two or more events. The significance of the interaction of intervention and shift or intervention, shift, and block was the important question in our study. After significance of an interaction is obtained, Bakeman suggests the adjusted residual (Haberman 1978) for the cells involved in the interaction. These adjusted residuals provide a way of obtaining a probability for each cell, and this probability indicates which cells contribute to the overall significance (note that in 2×2 tables all four adjusted residuals have the same absolute value, indicating equivalence or equal contributions). Adjusted residuals compare the actual observed frequency in a particular cell of the contingency table (which gives the frequency of presence or absence of the intervention with a particular category of shift) with the expected frequency that would be obtained solely by chance. These expected or chance frequencies are a function of the base rate for presence of an intervention and the base rate for the various categories of shifts. If the base rate for either the intervention or a category of shift is particularly low, it is especially important to take account of what would be expected by chance alone. It is difficult without a statistical test to identify those cells where the actual observed frequencies are considerably more or less than what would be expected by chance alone when base rates are low for either intervention or category of shift.

Our first hierarchical analysis considered two dimensions: 1) presence or absence of a particular intervention and 2) four categories of shift in collaboration. The interventions analyzed (in separate analyses) were relationship or transference (R), interpretation (I), and interpretation focused on relationship (IR). The second kind of hierarchical analysis was three dimensional with intervention, shift, and session block (early, middle, late) as the dimensions. In some analyses, shift in collaboration was considered as having only two categories: positive shift or negative shift.

The analyses were considered as exploratory with no specific hypotheses about the pattern of a relationship between intervention and shift. A limitation imposed by the method is the inability to include the absence of a shift. To use this kind of sequential analysis with our data, one of the events must be identified as the target event, either antecedent or consequent, and the other event then recorded for a given lag. In our study, we identified the presence of a shift as the target event, in this case the consequent event, and then looked back through all interventions, at most 50 lines prior to the given target event but not including the preceding target event, to see if a particular intervention had occurred. If an intervention of the type under consideration occurred, this was tallied opposite the proper category of shift. This procedure was continued until all shifts were included.

Results

Mr. Black

The results of the statistical tests using a two-dimensional hierarchical model for the R intervention are presented first. The interaction term (intervention × shift) was significant ($P = .0518$).

Analysis of the adjusted residuals (see Table C–1) showed that only two cells made a significant contribution to the overall significant interaction term. These were the cells in which the observed frequency of positive partial shifts was significantly greater than the expected frequency (8 versus 5.1) when there was not an R intervention and the cell in which the observed frequency of positive partial shifts was significantly less than the expected frequency (8 versus 10.9) when there was an R intervention. Although the observed frequency of positive shifts was larger than the expected frequency when there was an R intervention, and the observed frequency of positive partial shifts was smaller than expected when there was not an R intervention, neither of the adjusted residuals for these cells reached significance.

Thinking that breaking down shift in collaboration into four categories, which distinguished between partial and full shifts, might be too fine a categorization, we next analyzed the two-dimensional model with shift categorized as either positive or negative. Again, the interaction term was significant ($P = .0146$). Examination of the adjusted residuals, which are identical in absolute value for all four cells, revealed a significant contribution ($P = .0456$) in all four cells. When there was no R intervention, there were more positive shifts than expected by chance (14 versus 11.8) and fewer negative shifts than expected by chance (0 versus 2.2). When there was an R intervention, there were fewer positive shifts than expected (23 versus 25.2) and more negative shifts than expected (7 versus 4.8).

Table C-1. Contingency table, expected (chance) frequencies, adjusted residuals, and probability for intervention R: Mr. Black

	Four-dimensional model				Two-dimensional model		
	Negative shifts	Negative partial shifts	Positive partial shifts	Positive shifts	Negative shifts	Positive shifts	Number of shifts
No R							
Observed frequency	0	0	8	6	0	14	14
Expected frequency	1.0	1.3	5.1	6.7	2.2	11.8	
Adjusted residuals	-1.2	-1.4	2.0	-0.4	-2.0	2.0	
P	NS	NS	.0456	NS	.0456	.0456	
R							
Observed frequency	3	4	8	15	7	23	30
Expected frequency	2.0	2.7	10.9	14.3	4.8	25.2	
Adjusted residuals	1.2	1.4	-2.0	0.4	2.0	-2.0	
P	NS	NS	.0456	NS	.0456	.0456	
Number of shifts	3	4	16	21	7	37	44

Next, we tested the three-dimensional model with R as the intervention, four-category shift, and block (early, middle, and late sessions) as the third dimension. Only the interaction of intervention and shift was significant.

Results were completely identical to the two-dimensional analysis. Block was not significant alone or in any interaction.

Next, the intervention I was analyzed with four-category shift. The interaction of intervention and shift was nonsignificant. The analysis of the intervention IR with a four-category shift yielded a nonsignificant interaction.

Results for Mr. Black were consistent in that interventions I and IR did not interact significantly with shift regardless of the number of categories of shift. Consistent results were obtained for intervention R, for which the interaction was significant regardless of whether four- or two-category shift was used. When there was no R intervention, there were more positive partial shifts than expected, and fewer positive partial shifts than expected when there was an R intervention. When positive full shifts and positive partial shifts were combined and there was no R intervention, there were more positive shifts than expected and fewer negative shifts than expected. When there was an R intervention, there were fewer positive shifts than expected and more negative shifts than expected.

For Mr. Black, the 44 shifts were almost entirely positive— 21 positive shifts and 16 positive partial shifts as opposed to only 3 negative shifts and 4 negative partial shifts. This disproportionate distribution of shifts may have limited the results of the analysis.

Ms. Green

The results with a two-dimensional hierarchical model using R as the intervention and four-category shift were that the interaction tended toward significance ($P = .0817$).

Adjusted residuals showed a trend toward significant contributions ($P = .0574$) for only two cells. There was a tendency toward fewer negative partial shifts than expected by chance (1 versus 3.2) when there was no R interaction and a tendency toward more negative partial shifts than expected by chance (6 versus 3.8) where there was an R intervention. Neither positive partial shifts nor positive shifts exceeded what was expected when there was an R intervention, and neither of the adjusted residuals for these cells was statistically significant, indicating that the actual frequencies of partial and full positive shifts when there was an R intervention did not differ from what could be expected by chance (Table C–2).

In the analysis of intervention I with four-category shift, the interaction was not significant. Similarly, in the analysis with IR as intervention and four-category shift, the interaction was not significant.

All three intervention analyses were repeated using two-category shift. For I and IR, the interaction term was again not significant. Although the results for the R intervention tended toward significance with four-category shift, the interaction became significant ($P = .0209$) with two-category shift. All adjusted residuals (identical in absolute value for all four cells) were significant ($P = .0278$). There were fewer negative shifts than expected (2 versus 5) and more positive shifts than expected (12 versus 9) when there was no R intervention and more negative shifts than expected (9 versus 6) and fewer positive shifts than expected when there was an R intervention.

Results were consistent for Ms. Green for either four- or two-category shift. There were considerably fewer shifts for Ms. Green than for Mr. Black, and there was a strange distribution of four-category shift—15 positive partial shifts but only 5 positive shifts, and 7 negative partial shifts but only 4 negative shifts. Although the proportion of negative and positive shifts was nearly equal for Ms. Green, the preponderance of partial shifts as compared with full shifts may have limited the results of the four-category shift analyses.

Ms. White

Analyses were conducted for Ms. White using interventions R, I, and IR successively and four-category shift. In all these analyses, the interaction was not significant. When two-category shift was used, inspection of the contingency tables indicated that analyses of these tables would not change the results from those obtained with four-category shift. Examination of the tables for either four- or two-category shift showed that the expected frequencies were extremely close to the actual frequencies in the cells. This implied that the actual

Table C–2. Contingency table, expected (chance) frequencies, adjusted residuals, and probability for intervention R: Ms. Green

	Four-dimensional model				Two-dimensional model		
	Negative shifts	Negative partial shifts	Positive partial shifts	Positive shifts	Negative shifts	Positive shifts	Number of shifts
No R							
Observed frequency	1	1	8	4	2	12	14
Expected frequency	1.8	3.2	6.8	2.3	5.0	9.0	
Adjusted residuals	−0.9	−1.9	0.9	1.7	−2.2	2.2	
P	NS	.0574	NS	NS	.0278	.0278	
R							
Observed frequency	3	6	7	1	9	8	17
Expected frequency	2.2	3.8	8.2	2.7	6.0	11.0	
Adjusted residuals	0.9	1.9	−0.9	−1.7	2.2	−2.2	
P	NS	.0574	NS	NS	.0278	.0278	
Number of shifts	4	7	15	5	11	20	31

distribution of frequencies in the cells describing the interaction of intervention and shift followed approximately what could be expected by chance. Thus, no further analyses were conducted for Ms. White.

The results for Ms. White were very consistent; the interaction was nonsignificant regardless of the intervention or the number of categories of shift used. Ms. White had even fewer shifts (26) than Mr. Black (44) or Ms. Green (31), and the number of negative shifts was particularly low, 1 negative shift and 6 negative partial shifts. There were 7 positive partial shifts and 12 positive shifts. Both the small number of shifts and the disproportionate low number of negative shifts likely limited the results of the analyses.

Discussion

For Mr. Black, when four-category shift was used, there were significantly fewer positive partial shifts than expected by chance when there was an R intervention and significantly more positive partial shifts than expected when there was no R intervention. There were more positive full shifts than expected when there was an R intervention and fewer positive full shifts than expected when there was no R intervention, but neither of these reached significance. When two-category shift was used—that is, when partial and full shifts were combined for both negative and positive shifts—there were fewer total positive shifts than expected and more total negative shifts than expected when there was an R intervention, and more total positive shifts than expected and fewer total negative shifts than expected when there was no R intervention. All together, there is some evidence that R is a high-risk intervention and weaker evidence that it also is a high-gain intervention; that is, an R intervention may produce either positive or negative shifts in collaboration with the odds less in favor of positive shifts.

Mr. Black had the most shifts (44) in his 17 sessions (which ranged from session 16 to session 728). Of the shifts, 84% were positive, either partial or full shifts. Of those shifts (positive or negative), 68% followed (within 50 lines) an R intervention.

For Ms. Green, using four-category shift, there were more negative partial shifts than expected by chance when there was an R intervention and fewer negative partial shifts than expected when there was no R intervention. When partial and full shifts were collapsed, there were more total negative shifts than expected and fewer total positive shifts than expected when there was an R intervention, and fewer total negative shifts than expected and more total positive shifts than expected when there was no R intervention. There were not more positive shifts than expected by chance when there was an R intervention. Thus, for Ms. Green, R seems to be more of a high-risk intervention. Even inspection of the observed frequencies supports this, because there were 8 (47%) total positive shifts following an R intervention and 9 (53%) total negative shifts following an R intervention.

Ms. Green had 31 shifts in her 18 sessions (which ranged from session 4 to session 163). Of the total positive shifts for Ms. Green, 75% were positive partial shifts, and 64% of the total negative shifts were negative partial shifts. There were 65% total positive shifts. Of the shifts (positive or negative), 55% followed an R intervention.

For Ms. White, there were no significant relationships between intervention and shift, either four-category or two-category. The patterning of shift categories and presence or absence of an intervention very closely approximated what could be expected by chance. There were only 26 shifts for Ms. White in her 18 sessions (which ranged from session 6 to session 144). Of the shifts, 73% were positive, either partial or full shifts; 77% (either positive or negative) followed an R intervention.

Because log linear analysis analyzes discrete or category data using a type of chi-square test (likelihood ratio chi-square), which is a nonparametric test less powerful than parametric statistical tests, and sample sizes were only 44, 31, and 26, respectively, power has undoubtedly been limited in all of the analyses described. In addition, for chi-square tests, the ability to detect significant relationships is maximal when the marginal frequencies for presence or absence of an intervention and four- or two-category shifts are approximately equal. For all three patients, and particularly for Mr. Black and Ms. White, positive shifts, either partial or full, predominated—fortunate for the therapy but not for a relationship between shift and intervention to emerge. Similarly limiting the ability for a relationship to emerge was the predominance of R interventions preceding any shift for

Mr. Black and Ms. White. In all three cases with disproportionate numbers of positive shifts versus negative shifts and R interventions versus no R interventions, interpretation based on only observed frequencies can be problematic.

In addition to the power limitations in this study, there are at least two design limitations. The use of 50 lines prior to a shift is to some extent an arbitrary decision. The investigators thought that it was not appropriate to consider only the last intervention preceding the shift because they believed that the effect of a particular intervention might be delayed; thus, 50 lines prior to the shift was an estimate of the maximum amount of time that a shift following a particular intervention might be delayed. It is possible that different results would have been obtained if a different definition had been used.

Probably the most important limitation imposed by the design was the inability to include absence of shift as a category of shift, because we defined shift as the target event and then looked for an intervention as the antecedent event. Thus, the dimension of shift does not contain a zero category between the negative and positive categories. It seems likely that the presence of a no-shift category would have increased the ability for a relationship to emerge, because the total number of observations would have been based on interventions rather than on shifts and would have been considerably larger than the sample sizes in the analyses reported. The shift categories would then represent a true continuum, and a more complete pattern of relationships (either linear or nonlinear) would be possible.

The use of Bakeman's sequential analysis method, log linear analysis, and tests of the adjusted residuals was an exploratory attempt to provide a statistical test of the relationship between presence or absence of an intervention and ordered categories of shifts in collaboration, both only category data. Although the observations that were tallied represented a time dimension to a certain extent, there were irregularities in this time dimension. Observations were collected within a session, and pairs and triplets of successive sessions were included, but moderate to very large gaps between the pairs and triplets of sessions were present for all three patients. These irregularities precluded the use of various time series analyses, which have been recommended for controlled single-case studies.

References

Bakeman R: Untangling streams of behavior: sequential analysis of observation data, in Observing Behavior, Vol 2: Data Collection and Analysis Methods. Edited by Sackett GP. Baltimore, MD, University Park Press, 1978, pp 63–78

Bakeman R: Computing lag sequential statistics: the ELAG program. Behavior Research Methods and Instrumentation 15:530–535, 1983

Bakeman R, Gottman J: Observing Interaction: An Introduction to Sequential Analysis. Cambridge, UK, Cambridge University Press, 1986

Bishop Y, Fienberg S, Holland P: Discrete Multivariate Analysis. Cambridge, MA, The MIT Press, 1975

Haberman S: Analysis of Qualitative Data, Vol 1: Introductory Topics. New York, Academic Press, 1978, pp 77–79

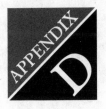

Quantitative Data

This appendix contains tables providing 1) the assessment of levels of functioning, 2) the intervention consensus ratings profiles, 3) the contribution of therapist's interventions to shifts in collaboration, and 4) the consensus of ratings on the Bellak Scales of Ego Functions—all for Mr. Black, Ms. Green, and Ms. White.

Table D–1. Assessing levels of functioning, baseline and outcome: Mr. Black

	1 2 3	4 5	6 7
Ego function	Active pursuit of stable goals. Tolerates frustration and maintains motivation in pursuit of goals. Defenses primarily obsessional, subliminative, repressive.	Sets stable goals but pursuit deflected by moderate degree of frustration. Undermines positive pursuits and assumes passive stance under stress. Lapses into use of primitive defenses.	Intolerant of frustration; unable to pursue stable goals. Passive, entitled stance; refuses responsibility for own welfare. Reliance on denial, projection, splitting.
Behavior	Absence of purposeful self-destructive behavior. Productive in vocational role, stable social ties. Affects appropriate in intensity and to situation; range includes guilt and humor.	Self-destructive behavior, ego-dystonic but persists sporadically. Impulsive/disruptive of social and vocational roles under stress. Lapses into inappropriate anger, disabling depression.	Actively self-destructive. Unable to maintain stable institutional ties; poor work history. Affects inappropriate in social context and intensity; rage and depression predominate.

Ego function: baseline marked (X) at 2; outcome circled at 4.

Behavior: baseline marked (X) at 2; outcome circled near 3–4.

	1	2	3	4	5	6	7
Object relations	Durable, stable intimate relations. Tolerant and sensitive to needs of others. Not particularly exploitative or controlling.		Limited capacity for intimacy. Some ability to sense and tolerate needs of others. Continued reliance on manipulation to control important others.		Chaotic and short-lived relationships. Hostile-dependent and superficial object ties. Requires absolute control to sustain relationships.		
Sense of self	Clear and stable sense of identity that does not vacillate with circumstance. Has appropriate sense of own strengths and limitations. Able to be alone comfortably.		Fragile sense of self; moderate suggestibility. Stress prompts flight into grandiosity or self-hatred. Ability to tolerate being alone for limited periods of time.		Little sense of identity; beliefs and self-concept vacillate widely with circumstance. Grandiosity coexists/alternates with low self-esteem and self-denigration. Cannot tolerate being alone.		

Note. Circled number indicates patient's level of functioning before treatment. Number crossed out indicates patient's level of functioning at follow-up.
Source. Scale from Waldinger and Gunderson 1987, with permission.

Table D–2.   Intervention consensus ratings profiles: Mr. Black

Session	Type of intervention							Nontransference versus transference		Expressive-supportive ratings	
	Interpretation	Confrontation	Clarification	Encouragement to elaborate	Affirmation	Empathy	Advice & praise	Nontransference	Transference	Expressive	Supportive
16	8	1	2	6	1	0	0	6	11	6	3
22	7	1	2	5	0	0	0	5	10	6	3
114	9	1	2	9	0	0	0	12	9	5	2
115	6	6	0	10	1	0	3	10	15	6	3
194	6	3	7	8	7	0	1	8	17	6	2
195	8	3	4	13	6	0	0	10	18	6	2
309	2	4	5	12	8	0	1	9	15	6	3
310	4	4	1	11	32	0	0	5	15	6	2
404	3	1	4	8	0	0	0	3	13	5	2
405	5	2	1	6	0	0	0	9	5	6	2
526	6	4	8	5	2	0	0	19	4	5	3
527	2	0	5	7	3	0	0	12	2	5	3
604	4	1	11	15	25	0	0	22	9	5	3
605	5	3	3	6	0	0	1	11	7	5	3
726	4	1	2	14	25	0	0	16	5	6	3
727	4	4	5	6	39	0	1	9	11	5	3
728	5	5	3	7	18	0	0	12	8	6	2

Table D–3. Contribution of therapist's interventions to shifts in collaboration: Mr. Black

Session and shift	Direction of shift	Therapist intervention viewed as contributory?	Coding of contributory interventions[a]	Comments
Session 16				
1	PS+	Yes	IR, IR	
2	S+	Yes	ER	
Session 22				
1	PS+	Yes	ER, ER	
2	S+	Yes	IR	
Session 114				
1	S+	Unclear	—	
Session 115				
1	PS+	Yes	U	
2	S+	Yes	CR, IR, IR	
3	S+	Yes	CR, APR	
4	PS-	Yes	CR	
5	S-	Yes	CR	
6	S+	Yes	CR, IR	
Session 194				
1	PS+	Unclear	—	Spontaneous reference to transference reflects his having internalized the expectations of transference (applies to shifts 1 & 2).
2	S+	Unclear	—	
3	PS+	Yes	IR	
Session 195				
1	PS+	Unclear	—	Transference established an encouraging, accepting climate.
2	PS+	Yes	IX	
3	S+	Yes	IR	
4	PS+	Unclear	—	Cumulative effort of prior interventions.

(continued)

Table D–3. Contribution of therapist's interventions to shifts in collaboration: Mr. Black *(continued)*

Session and shift	Direction of shift	Therapist intervention viewed as contributory?	Coding of contributory interventions[a]	Comments
Session 309				
1	PS+	Yes	EX, EX	
2	S+	Yes	CR, CR	
3	S+	Yes	ER, APR	
4	S–	Unclear	—	Difference of opinion.
Session 310				
1	PS+	Yes	ER	
2	PS–	Unclear	—	Divided opinion.
3	S–	Yes	ER	Some felt this intervention led to a positive shift after initial downward shift.
Session 404				
1	S+	Yes	ER, ER, CLR	
Session 405				
1	PS+	Yes	EX	
2	S+	Yes	IX	
3	PS+	Unclear	—	Patient apparently reacts to his own associations.
4	S+	Yes	IR, CX	
Session 526				
1	PS+	No	—	
2	S+	Yes	EX	A nontransference intervention facilitated affective communication; patient was too threatened to deal with transference hostility.
3	PS–	Yes	IR	Too direct, confrontive, unempathic, and too long.
Session 527				
1	S+	Yes	CLX	
2	PS+	Yes	CLX	
3	S+	Unclear	—	

Table D–3. Contribution of therapist's interventions to shifts in collaboration: Mr. Black *(continued)*

Session and shift	Direction of shift	Therapist intervention viewed as contributory?	Coding of contributory interventions[a]	Comments
Session 604				
1	S+	Yes	ER, ER	
Session 605				
1	S+	Yes	EX, CR	
2	S+	Yes	IX	
Session 726				
1	PS+	Yes	CLX and cumulative impact	
2	S+	Yes	IR, IR	
3	PS-	Unclear	—	
Session 727				
1	S+	Yes	CLR	
2	PS+	Yes	IR	
Session 728				
1	S+	Yes	IR and persistent backdrop of clarifying in a nonthreatening way the patient's feelings about termination.	
2	PS+	Unclear	—	Earlier clarification about acting out may have helped.
3	PS+	Yes	IR	
4	PS+	Yes	CR	

[a]Explanation of coding categories:
APR = Advice and/or praise of adaptive behavior focusing on the therapeutic situation.
CR = Confrontation with aspects of therapeutic experience.
CX = Confrontation with aspects of extratherapy experience.
IR = Interpretation of transference.
IX = Interpretation of extratransference.
CLR = Clarification/restatement of patient's wording with regard to therapeutic situations.
CLX = Clarification/restatement of patient's wording with regard to extratherapy situations.
ER = Encouragement to elaborate on therapeutic experience.
EX = Encouragement to elaborate on extratherapy experience.

Table D–4. Consensus of ratings on the Bellak Scales of Ego Functions: Mr. Black

	Initial	Outcome
Reality testing	6.0	6.5
Judgment	4.5	5.5
Regulation and control	3.5	5.0
Object relations		
Degree and kind of relatedness	4.0	5.0
Primitivity-maturity	4.0	4.5
Responsiveness to others	4.0	5.5
Object constancy	3.0	5.5
Thought processes	6.0	6.5
Defensive functioning		
Adaptive level	4.0	5.5
Success-failure	3.0	5.5
Autonomous functioning	5.0	6.5
Synthetic-integrative functioning	4.5	6.0
Mastery-competence	4.0	6.5
Superego adaptation	3.0	5.0

Table D-5. Assessing levels of functioning, baseline and outcome: Ms. Green

	1	2	3	4	5	6	7
Ego function	Active pursuit of stable goals. Tolerates frustration and maintains motivation in pursuit of goals. Defenses primarily obsessional, subliminative, repressive.		✗	Sets stable goals but pursuit deflected by moderate degree of frustration. Undermines positive pursuits and assumes passive stance under stress. Lapses into use of primitive defenses.		⑥ Intolerant of frustration; unable to pursue stable goals. Passive, entitled stance; refuses responsibility for own welfare. Reliance on denial, projection, splitting.	
Behavior	Absence of purposeful self-destructive behavior. Productive in vocational role, stable social ties. Affects appropriate in intensity and to situation; range includes guilt and humor.		✗	Self-destructive behavior, ego-dystonic but persists sporadically. Impulsive/disruptive of social and vocational roles under stress. Lapses into inappropriate anger, disabling depression.	①	Actively self-destructive. Unable to maintain stable institutional ties; poor work history. Affects inappropriate in social context and intensity; rage and depression predominate.	

(continued)

Table D–5. Assessing levels of functioning, baseline and outcome: Ms. Green (*continued*)

	1	2	3	4	5	6	7
Object relations	Durable, stable intimate relations. Tolerant and sensitive to needs of others. Not particularly exploitative or controlling.		Limited capacity for intimacy. Some ability to sense and tolerate needs of others. Continued reliance on manipulation to control important others.		✗	⊖	Chaotic and short-lived relationships. Hostile-dependent and superficial object ties. Requires absolute control to sustain relationships.
Sense of self	Clear and stable sense of identity that does not vacillate with circumstance. Has appropriate sense of own strengths and limitations. Able to be alone comfortably.		Fragile sense of self; moderate suggestibility. Stress prompts flight into grandiosity or self-hatred. Ability to tolerate being alone for limited periods of time.	✗		⊖	Little sense of identity; beliefs and self-concept vacillate widely with circumstance. Grandiosity coexists/alternates with low self-esteem and self-denigration. Cannot tolerate being alone.

Note. Circled number indicates patient's level of functioning before treatment. Number crossed out indicates patient's level of functioning at follow-up.

Source. Scale from Waldinger and Gunderson 1987, with permission.

Table D-6. Intervention consensus ratings profiles: Ms. Green

| Session | Type of intervention | | | | | | | Nontransference versus transference ratings | | Expressive-supportive ratings | |
	Interpre-tation	Confron-tation	Clari-fication	Encourage-ment to elaborate	Affir-mation	Empathy	Advice & praise	Nontrans-ference	Trans-ference	Expressive	Supportive
4	5	11	19	28	1	1	0	53	11	4	4
5	6	13	14	46	4	0	1	65	15	4	4
6	8	25	16	44	15	0	1	74	20	4	4
30	6	27	6	20	6	2	3	52	12	4	6
31	11	22	21	58	38	0	0	101	11	5	4
32	2	26	20	53	34	1	0	87	15	5	4
59	2	37	6	29	7	0	19	93	0	3	6
60	10	22	10	51	57	2	0	79	16	5	4
61	1	24	3	35	8	0	23	79	7	3	5
88	5	9	15	32	3	0	1	42	20	5	4
89	3	17	11	29	1	0	2	38	24	5	3
90	10	11	6	25	8	0	2	34	20	6	3
129	0	15	11	23	56	0	12	58	3	3	5
130	5	24	8	31	58	2	9	70	9	4	5
131	0	9	3	51	107	1	10	73	1	4	4
161	0	4	3	17	5	4	2	30	0	2	6
162	0	22	4	32	37	0	0	52	6	4	4
163	1	17	8	28	54	1	3	56	2	4	5

Table D–7. Contribution of therapist's interventions to shifts in collaboration: Ms. Green

Session and shift	Direction of shift	Therapist intervention viewed as contributory?	Coding of contributory interventions[a]	Comments
Session 4				
1	S+	Yes	IR, CLX, EX	Empathic, non-critical series.
Session 5				
1	S+	Yes	EX	Gentle, noncritical inquiries.
2	PS+	Yes	CLX	Interest, empathy, desire to be helpful.
Session 6				
1	PS+	Yes	CX	Steady, mildly confrontive.
2	PS+	Yes	CR, CR	Firmly keeping focus on patient's distrust.
3	PS+	Yes	IR	Persistent trans-ference focus.
Session 30				
1	S–	Yes	CX, CX	Patient left session early in a state of anger.
Session 31				
1	S+	Yes	EX, CLX	Close tracking of patient.
2	S–	Yes	CR	Pursues transference.
3	PS+	Yes	CR, CX, IX, IR	Pursues response to absence.
4	PS–	Yes	CX	
Session 32				
1	PS+	Yes	EX	Focus on fearfulness.
2	PS–	Yes	CR	Focus on anger.
Session 59				
1	S+	Yes	CX, IX, CX, APX	Many interventions repeatedly and unequivocally take the side of the patient staying in treatment.

Table D–7. Contribution of therapist's interventions to shifts in collaboration: Ms. Green (continued)

Session and shift	Direction of shift	Therapist intervention viewed as contributory?	Coding of contributory interventions[a]	Comments
Session 60				
1	PS+	Climate	—	Neutrality in response to provocation.
2	PS+	Yes	CLX, CX	Accepting, empathic inquiry.
Session 61				
1	PS+	Spontaneous	—	Persistent effort to encourage reflectiveness while failing to be intimidated.
Session 88				
1	PS–	Unclear	—	
Session 89				
No shifts				
Session 90				
1	PS+	Yes	CLX	Listening and empathy.
2	S–	Yes	IX	Implied criticism of patient.
3	PS+	Yes	CR	Persistence in addressing patient's anger.
Session 129				
1	PS+	Yes	CX, EX	Support and persistence.
2	PS+	Yes	CX	Gentle and supportive focus on anger with boyfriend.
3	S+	Yes	APX	Casts her angry behavior in a positive light.
Session 130				
No shifts				

(continued)

Table D–7. Contribution of therapist's interventions to shifts in collaboration: Ms. Green *(continued)*

Session and shift	Direction of shift	Therapist intervention viewed as contributory?	Coding of contributory interventions[a]	Comments
Session 131				
1	PS+	Yes	EX	
2	PS–	No	—	
3	PS–	Yes	EX, EX	
Session 161				
1	S–	Yes	CX, CX	Efforts to encourage reflection are in vain.
Session 162				
1	PS–	Yes	CX	Focus on patient's "failure"—implied criticism.
Session 163				
1	PS–	Unclear	—	
2	PS+	Yes	CLX, CX, CX, CX	Concerted and persistent effort.

[a]Explanation of coding categories:
APR = Advice and/or praise of adaptive behavior focusing on the therapeutic situation.
CR = Confrontation with aspects of therapeutic experience.
CX = Confrontation with aspects of extratherapy experience.
IR = Interpretation of transference.
IX = Interpretation of extratransference.
CLR = Clarification/restatement of patient's wording with regard to therapeutic situations.
CLX = Clarification/restatement of patient's wording with regard to extratherapy situations.
ER = Encouragement to elaborate on therapeutic experience.
EX = Encouragement to elaborate on extratherapy experience.

Table D–8. Consensus of ratings on the Bellak Scales of Ego Functions: Ms. Green

	Initial	Outcome
Reality testing	4.0	5.0
Judgment	2.5	4.0
Regulation and control	2.5	4.0
Object relations		
Degree and kind of relatedness	2.5	3.5
Primitivity-maturity	3.0	3.5
Responsiveness to others	2.5	3.5
Object constancy	3.0	3.0
Thought processes	3.5	4.0
Defensive functioning		
Adaptive level	2.0	4.0
Success-failure	3.0	4.0
Autonomous functioning	2.5	4.5
Synthetic-integrative functioning	2.5	4.0
Mastery-competence	2.0	4.5
Superego adaptation	3.0	4.0

Table D–9. Assessing levels of functioning, baseline and outcome: Ms. White

Ego function

Scale: 1 2 (✗) 3 (①) 4 5 6 7

- **(1–2)** Active pursuit of stable goals. Tolerates frustration and maintains motivation in pursuit of goals. Defenses primarily obsessional, subliminative, repressive.
- **(4–5)** Sets stable goals but pursuit deflected by moderate degree of frustration. Undermines positive pursuits and assumes passive stance under stress. Lapses into use of primitive defenses.
- **(6–7)** Intolerant of frustration; unable to pursue stable goals. Passive, entitled stance; refuses responsibility for own welfare. Reliance on denial, projection, splitting.

Behavior

Scale: 1 2 (✗) 3 4 (④) 5 6 7

- **(1–2)** Absence of purposeful self-destructive behavior. Productive in vocational role, stable social ties. Affects appropriate in intensity and to situation; range includes guilt and humor.
- **(4–5)** Self-destructive behavior, ego-dystonic but persists sporadically. Impulsive/disruptive of social and vocational roles under stress. Lapses into inappropriate anger, disabling depression.
- **(6–7)** Actively self-destructive. Unable to maintain stable institutional ties; poor work history. Affects inappropriate in social context and intensity; rage and depression predominate.

	1	2	3	4	5	6	7
Object relations	Durable, stable intimate relations. Tolerant and sensitive to needs of others. Not particularly exploitative or controlling.	⊗	①	Limited capacity for intimacy. Some ability to sense and tolerate needs of others. Continued reliance on manipulation to control important others.		Chaotic and short-lived relationships. Hostile-dependent and superficial object ties. Requires absolute control to sustain relationships.	
Sense of self	Clear and stable sense of identity that does not vacillate with circumstance. Has appropriate sense of own strengths and limitations. Able to be alone comfortably.	⊗		Fragile sense of self; moderate suggestibility. Stress prompts flight into grandiosity or self-hatred. Ability to tolerate being alone for limited periods of time. ①		Little sense of identity; beliefs and self-concept vacillate widely with circumstance. Grandiosity coexists/alternates with low self-esteem and self-denigration. Cannot tolerate being alone.	

Note.   Circled number indicates patient's level of functioning before treatment. Number crossed out indicates patient's level of functioning at follow-up.
Source.   Scale from Waldinger and Gunderson 1987, with permission.

Table D-10. Intervention consensus ratings profiles: Ms. White

	Type of intervention							Nontransference versus transference		Expressive-supportive ratings	
Session	Interpretation	Confrontation	Clarification	Encouragement to elaborate	Affirmation	Empathy	Advice & praise	Nontransference	Transference	Expressive	Supportive
6	3	2	2	11	12	1	6	7	18	5	4
7	2	4	2	16	1	0	2	14	12	5	3
8	8	3	1	15	2	0	1	14	14	5	4
30	0	8	0	14	8	0	0	6	16	6	3
31	0	6	0	11	2	0	0	10	7	6	3
32	0	4	0	14	4	0	0	13	5	6	2
55	4	8	1	4	1	0	0	1	16	6	2
56	2	3	1	21	8	0	0	5	22	5	3
57	6	6	0	14	9	1	1	3	25	6	3
89	6	4	0	6	0	0	0	5	11	6	3
90	3	5	0	2	1	0	10	10	10	5	5
91	8	5	1	23	8	1	7	26	19	5	6
121	1	2	2	21	15	0	0	12	14	6	3
122	5	6	0	8	5	0	0	9	10	5	3
123	1	3	4	12	2	0	0	14	6	5	3
142	5	6	0	7	5	0	0	8	10	6	3
143	0	7	0	14	4	0	0	13	8	6	3
144	5	10	1	12	8	0	1	15	14	6	3

Table D–11. Contribution of therapist's interventions to shifts in collaboration: Ms. White

Session and shift	Direction of shift	Therapist intervention viewed as contributory?	Coding of contributory interventions[a]	Comments
Session 6				
1	S+	Yes	ER, EX	
2	S+	Yes	IR	
Session 7				
1	S+	Yes	CX, EX	
2	S+	Yes	CR	The shift was influenced by a cumulative effect of interventions.
Session 8				
1	PS+	Yes	IR	Series of other interventions also contributed to the shift.
2	PS–	Yes	IR	
Session 30				
1	PS+	Yes	CR	The shift was influenced by a cumulative effect of interventions.
Session 31				
No shifts				
Session 32				
1	S+	Yes	EX	Series of other interventions also contributed to the shift.
Session 55				
1	PS–	Yes	CR, CR	
2	S+	Yes	IR	The shift was influenced by a cumulative effect of interventions.

(continued)

Table D–11. Contribution of therapist's interventions to shifts in collaboration: Ms. White *(continued)*

Session and shift	Direction of shift	Therapist intervention viewed as contributory?	Coding of contributory interventions[a]	Comments
Session 56				
1	S+	Yes	IR	
2	PS–	Unclear	Unclear	Therapist interventions may have influenced the shift but more likely it was spontaneous due to patient's anger.
Session 57				
1	PS–	No	—	Spontaneous due to anger over interruptions of therapy.
2	PS+	Yes	IR	
Session 89				
1	PS–	Yes	IR	
Session 90				
1	S+	Yes	APR, APR, APR	A series of other interventions also influenced the shift.
Session 91				
1	PS–	Yes	IX, IX	
2	PS+	Yes	EMR, IR	A series of other interventions also influenced the shift.
Session 121				
1	S+	Yes	EX	
Session 122				
1	S–	No	—	The shift was spontaneous with the patient beginning the session wanting to flee therapy.
Session 123				
1	PS+	Unclear	—	The shift appeared to be spontaneous.
2	S+	Yes	IR	

Table D–11. Contribution of therapist's interventions to shifts in collaboration: Ms. White *(continued)*

Session and shift	Direction of shift	Therapist intervention viewed as contributory?	Coding of contributory interventions[a]	Comments
Session 142				
1	PS–	Yes	CR	
Session 143				
1	PS+	No	—	The patient reflected on her emotional response to the therapist spontaneously.
2	S+	Yes	ER, ER	
Session 144				
1	S+	Yes	ER	

[a]Explanation of coding categories:
APR = Advice and/or praise of adaptive behavior focusing on the therapeutic situation.
CR = Confrontation with aspects of therapeutic experience.
CX = Confrontation with aspects of extratherapy experience.
IR = Interpretation of transference.
IX = Interpretation of extratransference.
CLR = Clarification/restatement of patient's wording with regard to therapeutic situations.
CLX = Clarification/restatement of patient's wording with regard to extratherapy situations.
ER = Encouragement to elaborate on therapeutic experience.
EX = Encouragement to elaborate on extratherapy experience.

Table D–12. Consensus of ratings on the Bellak Scales of Ego
Functions: Ms. White

	Initial	Outcome
Reality testing	6.0	6.0
Judgment	4.5	6.0
Regulation and control	3.5	5.0
Object relations		
Degree and kind of relatedness	3.5	5.0
Primitivity-maturity	4.0	5.0
Responsiveness to others	3.5	5.0
Object constancy	3.5	5.0
Thought processes	5.0	6.0
Defensive functioning		
Adaptive level	3.5	5.0
Success-failure	3.0	4.0
Autonomous functioning	5.0	6.0
Synthetic-integrative functioning	5.0	5.5
Mastery-competence	5.0	6.0
Superego adaptation	4.0	5.0

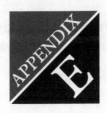

Manuals

Prediction Study Manual

Database

　　Initial case summary
　　Family history
　　Initial psychological test report
　　Videotape of initial Diagnostic Interview for Borderline
　　　　Patients
　　Transcripts of three early sessions
　　Bellak ratings at initial assessment (to be supplied by outcome
　　　　team)

Instructions

1. Please read over the enclosed questionnaire before examining the
   initial data.
2. After reviewing all of the initial data, proceed to answer the enclosed questions as fully as possible and without consulting the
   other judge.
3. When both judges have completed their independent assessments, they should meet and jointly fill out a consensus questionnaire.

Prediction Study
Amenability to Psychotherapy

		Unfavorable						Favorable			
1.	Friendliness	−5	−4	−3	−2	−1	1	2	3	4	5
				hostile					amiable		
2.	Likeability	−5	−4	−3	−2	−1	1	2	3	4	5
				below average					above average		
3.	Intelligence	−5	−4	−3	−2	−1	1	2	3	4	5
				below average					above average		
4.	Motivation	−5	−4	−3	−2	−1	1	2	3	4	5
				indifferent					motivated		
5.	Psychological-mindedness	−5	−4	−3	−2	−1	1	2	3	4	5
				low					high		
6.	Conscience factors	−5	−4	−3	−2	−1	1	2	3	4	5
			antisocial; deceitful; vengeful					values; good moral sense			
7.	Self-discipline	−5	−4	−3	−2	−1	1	2	3	4	5
				low; chaotic					high		
8.	Impulse control	−5	−4	−3	−2	−1	1	2	3	4	5
			craving; impulsivity						high		
9.	Defensive style	−5	−4	−3	−2	−1	1	2	3	4	5
				drugs; action					intrapunitive		
10.	Externalization/internalization	−5	−4	−3	−2	−1	1	2	3	4	5
				paranoid					capacity to admit fault		
11.	Empathy/narcissism	−5	−4	−3	−2	−1	1	2	3	4	5
			contempt; entitlement						ability to care about and resonate with others		
12.	Parental factors	−5	−4	−3	−2	−1	1	2	3	4	5
			brutalization; exploitation; indifference					warmth; support			
13.	Social supports	−5	−4	−3	−2	−1	1	2	3	4	5
				absent-disruptive					stable		

Closeness-Distance Description

We are interested in a detailed description of the person's mode of relating him- or herself to others with special attention to his or her pattern of closeness-seeking or distance-taking behaviors with regard to significant others. The pathological extreme of closeness seeking is seen in the individual who strives for symbiosis-merger, does not maintain firm boundaries between self and other, views the other as an extension of him- or herself, has difficulty in tolerating aloneness and separations, and has a low capacity for object constancy. The pathological extreme of distance taking is seen in the schizoid individual who is reclusive, avoids personal and social contacts, maintains an emotional barrier between self and others, and strives to be as self-sufficient as possible. The optimally healthy mode of relating is one in which emotional closeness and intimacy with a significant other is maintained in terms of being capable of communicating one's inner needs and feelings without losing sight of oneself or the other as a separate person. Also, the person is able to retain a sense of autonomy about him- or herself and is able to regulate his or her distance taking when appropriate. The description should include both a consideration of wishes and strivings as well as capacities to maintain certain behaviors.

1. To what extent does the patient strive for and achieve a mature emotional closeness to significant others in which appropriate boundaries are maintained between self and others?
2. To what extent does the patient strive for and maintain symbiotic-merger relations with significant others, including attention to patient's dependency wishes, magical expectations, and separation reactions?
3. To what extent does the patient strive for and maintain emotional distance from significant others? This includes the patient's need to withdraw from emotional contact with others; the patient's isolation from others; tendency to maintain superficial, as-if relationships; or emotional detachment.
4. To what extent does the patient fluctuate between a position of closeness and emotional relatedness on the one hand and with-

drawal and distance on the other? How extreme are these fluctuations? How much control and flexibility over closeness and distance regulation does the patient show?

Optimal Therapeutic Strategy

The following are the definitions of supportive and expressive treatment we are using.

Expressive treatment. The most expressive treatment is one that attempts to explore and uncover the patient's unconscious wishes, fears, conflicts, and defenses. The most potent means of achieving the goal of making the unconscious conscious is to explore the underlying difficulties in relationships, particularly the patient's relationship to the therapist. Toward this end, a variety of interventions, including encouragement to elaborate, clarification, and confrontation, may precede and work toward the explanatory formulation contained in an interpretation.

Supportive treatment. The supportive dimension is defined by those activities of the therapist/analyst that promote the patient's adaptive functioning both within and outside of the therapeutic interaction. The therapist's actions that facilitate the patient's functioning include the use of the person of the therapist as a source of emotional support, affirming adaptive behavior. As important, the therapist functions as a model for identification in which the therapist's reality testing, judgment, anticipation of consequences, emotional constraint, and appropriateness, as well as other ego functions, guide and structure the patient. Typical interventions that convey and promote the supportive actions of the therapist/analyst may involve advice, praise, empathic reactions, and the therapist's availability outside the regular appointments.

1. What are the main therapeutic issues you expect the patient to present over the course of the treatment?
2. Which issues, if any, should optimally be treated by expressive-uncovering techniques, including transference interpretation?
3. Which issues, if any, should optimally be treated by a more sup-

portive approach? What kind of supportive measures?

4. Would you anticipate shifts in treatment approaches during the course of the treatment and, if so, what kinds?

5. What are the characteristics of the patient that you regard as most relevant in determining your answers to the above questions?

6. Rate the optimal therapeutic strategy for this patient on the following supportiveness and expressiveness scales for the main part of the treatment.

Expressiveness:	1	2	3	4	5	6	7
	Very little or none			Moderate amount			Very much

Supportiveness:	1	2	3	4	5	6	7

Intervention Profile

1. Focus on the patient-therapist relationship versus nonrelationship (or transference versus nontransference).

   Please rate the optimal degree of emphasis or focus on the relationship versus the nonrelationship:

Patient-therapist relationship:	1	2	3	4	5	6	7
	No emphasis						Great emphasis

Nonrelationship:	1	2	3	4	5	6	7
	No emphasis						Great emphasis

2. Using the definitions provided for each intervention, write a sentence or two concerning the degree of emphasis that optimally should be placed on each intervention, including the basis for your judgment.

Interpretation. This consists of imparting to the patient the therapist's understanding of the unconscious motives, fears, or wishes that are embedded in the patient's verbalizations or behavior. The crucial attitude of an interpretation is that it must be explanatory.

Confrontation.   Confrontations either 1) deal with the patient's avoidance, minimization, or denial; or 2) *sharply underscore* an affect or content that the patient seems to be overlooking. Confrontations address something the patient does not want to accept or identifies the fact of the patient's avoidance or minimization.

Clarification.   A clarification consists of the therapist's summary, restatement, or reformulation of what the patient has said with significant changes that represent the therapist's effort *to convey a more coherent view* of what the patient has been attempting to describe.

Encouragement to elaborate.   This is broadly defined as a request for information about a topic already being discussed by the patient. Second, it could include the therapist's effort to select (focus) on a particular topic among several *that the patient has brought up.*

Affirmation.   This score is applied to simple affirmations—for example, "Um," "Um Hum," "Yeah," "I see," "Yes, I see what you mean."

Empathy.   This category demonstrates the therapist's attunement to the patient's emotional state. The scores should not be applied to delineations of specific contents, even though such comments may be made in an empathic manner.

Advice-praise.   This category includes *advice* to the patient regarding how best to proceed with or understand some aspect of his or her life or experience or with some aspect of treatment. *Praise* consists of recognizing, acknowledging, or commending the patient for an effort or achievement.

3. Rate each of these dimensions on a 7-point scale for optimal degrees of emphasis.

Interpretation:	1	2	3	4	5	6	7
	No emphasis		Little emphasis		Moderate emphasis		Great emphasis

Confrontation:	1	2	3	4	5	6	7

Clarification:	1	2	3	4	5	6	7

Encouragement to elaborate:	1	2	3	4	5	6	7

Affirmation:	1	2	3	4	5	6	7

Empathy:	1	2	3	4	5	6	7

Advice-praise:	1	2	3	4	5	6	7

Outcome Study Manual

I. Initial ratings
   A. Review initial data
      1. Case summary
      2. Family history
      3. Initial psychological test report
      4. Initial Diagnostic Interview for Borderline Patients
      5. Transcripts of first three sessions
   B. Rate (first do it independently, and then reach a consensus)
      1. Bellak Ego Function Assessment (EFA)
      2. Global Assessment Scale (GAS)
      3. Levels of Functioning
   C. Describe each of the following variables in a paragraph (first do it independently, and then reach a consensus)
      1. Core neurotic conflicts
      2. Self-concept
      3. Insight
      4. Psychological-mindedness
      5. Transference paradigms
II. Outcome ratings
   A. Review outcome data
      1. Discharge summary

      2. Termination psychological test report

      3. Termination Diagnostic Interview for Borderline Patients

      4. Transcripts of last three sessions

B. Rate (first do it independently)

      1. EFA

      2. GAS

C. Describe the *change* in the following variables (first do it independently)

      1. Core neurotic conflicts

      2. Self-concept

      3. Insight

      4. Psychological-mindedness

      5. Transference paradigms

D. Meet for consensus on B and C

E. Following the completion of the numerical ratings and narrative descriptions above, indicate in essay form those patient characteristics that you judge to be most influential in the outcome of the treatment

Treatment Interventions Project: Outcome Ratings

Patient number _____
Interval _____
Date of ratings _____

	Consensus	Judge 1	Judge 2
Bellak Ego Function Assessment (EFA)			
1. Reality testing	a.* ____	____	____
2. Judgment	a. ____	____	____
3. Regulation and control	b. ____	____	____
4. Object relations	a. ____	____	____
	b. ____	____	____
	c. ____	____	____
	d. ____	____	____
5. Thought processes	b. ____	____	____
6. Defensive functioning	a. ____	____	____
	b. ____	____	____
7. Autonomous functioning	b. ____	____	____
8. Synthetic-integrative functioning	b. ____	____	____
9. Mastery-competence	a. ____	____	____
10. Superego adaptation	a. ____	____	____
Global Assessment Scale	____	____	____

*The letters correspond to the sections of the Bellak EFA that were rated.

Outcome Study: Assessing Levels of Functioning: Baseline and Outcome

	1	2	3	4	5	6	7
Ego function	Active pursuit of stable goals.		Sets stable goals but pursuit deflected by moderate degree of frustration.			Intolerant of frustration; unable to pursue stable goals.	
	Tolerates frustration and maintains motivation in pursuit of goals.		Undermines positive pursuits and assumes passive stance under stress.			Passive, entitled stance; refuses responsibility for own welfare.	
	Defenses primarily obsessional, subliminative, repressive.		Lapses into use of primitive defenses.			Reliance on denial, projection, splitting.	
Behavior	Absence of purposeful self-destructive behavior.		Self-destructive behavior, ego-dystonic but persists sporadically.			Actively self-destructive.	
	Productive in vocational role, stable social ties.		Impulsive/disruptive of social and vocational roles under stress.			Unable to maintain stable institutional ties; poor work history.	
	Affects appropriate in intensity and to situation; range includes guilt and humor.		Lapses into inappropriate anger, disabling depression.			Affects inappropriate in social context and intensity; rage and depression predominate.	
Object relations	Durable, stable intimate relations.		Limited capacity for intimacy.			Chaotic and short-lived relationships.	
	Tolerant and sensitive to needs of others.		Some ability to sense and tolerate needs of others.			Hostile-dependent and superficial object ties.	
	Not particularly exploitative or controlling.		Continued reliance on manipulation to control important others.			Requires absolute control to sustain relationships.	

Sense of self	1	2	3	4	5	6	7
	Clear and stable sense of identity that does not vacillate with circumstance. Has appropriate sense of own strengths and limitations. Able to be alone comfortably.			Fragile sense of self; moderate suggestibility. Stress prompts flight into grandiosity or self-hatred. Ability to tolerate being alone for limited periods of time.		Little sense of identity; beliefs and self-concept vacillate widely with circumstance. Grandiosity coexists/alternates with low self-esteem and self-denigration. Cannot tolerate being alone.	

Source. Scale from Waldinger and Gunderson 1987.

Index